D0461778

Breathwalk

Breath**walk**

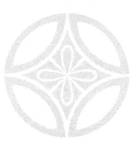

Breathing Your Way

to a Revitalized Body, Mind,

and Spirit

GURUCHARAN SINGH KHALSA, PH.D.,
AND YOGI BHAJAN, PH.D.

Foreword by Herbert Benson, M.D.

Broadway Books, New York

BROADWAY

Broadway Books titles may be purchased for business or promotional use or for special sales. For information, please write to: Special Markets Department, Random House, Inc., 1540 Broadway, New York, NY 10036.

BROADWAY BOOKS and its logo, a letter B bisected on the diagonal, are trademarks of Broadway Books, a division of Random House, Inc.

Visit our website at www.broadwaybooks.com

Library of Congress Cataloging-in-Publication Data
Khalsa, Gurucharan Singh.
Breathwalk: breathing your way to a revitalized body, mind, and spirit / by Gurucharan Singh Khalsa and Yogi Bhajan; foreword by Herbert Benson.—1st ed.
p. cm.
Includes bibliographical references and index.
1. Breathing exercises. 2. Fitness walking.
I. Bhajan, Yogi. II. Title.
RA782.K48 2000
613.7'176—dc21

99-087331

FIRST EDITION

Designed by Nicola Ferguson

ISBN 0-7679-0493-1

10 9 8 7 6 5 4 3 2 1

Kundalini
Research
Institute

This is dedicated to all those who wish to breathe new vitality and inspiration into their lives and into the lives of others, and to Guru Ram Das and all the teachers who have brought us this technology to live an exceptional and spirited life.

Contents

Contents

Contents

Foreword

I am happy to recommend Breathwalk to anyone who wants a simple method to improve his or her life. This book is written to help people help themselves. We all walk and breathe. Breathwalk adds focused attention and patterns of rhythmical breath and sound. This evokes the relaxation response and creates an immediate gateway to the cognitive and physiological potentials we all have within our mind/body interactions. Breathwalk is a way to exercise and increase our positive moods. It is an approach to access our innate powers of self-care. I have explored the process of healing and the scientific foundations for the use of evidence-based techniques, like meditation, for over thirty years. I am convinced of its applicability for all of us. We can each make simple choices to live a better and more fulfilled life.

I found in my research that there is a relaxation response produced by rhythmical exercise done with focused attention, as done in Breathwalk. Further, the benefits for positive mood elevation and enhanced healing are triggered by this combination and not just by exercise or walking alone.

Foreword

The Breathwalk as presented here by Yogi Bhajan and Gurucharan Khalsa has five steps. The first two, awaken and align, call attention to your body and to your walking form. The third step has intervals of rhythmical walking with breath control and a mental focus. This is a classical way to elicit the relaxation response. It is a fundamental way to open your mind for the cognitive restructuring that comes with effective healing. The use of what is called in this book "primal sounds"—a simple sound scale as you walk—helps to interrupt the constant chatter and static of the mind. In step four, balance, your mind often becomes very still and can open you to new emotional choices. Then, as the authors explain, if you choose to do the fifth step, the Innerwalk, you can direct your mind, remember your capability for wellness, and minimize any perceived inner conflicts. This sequence is an excellent way to exercise and to open your power to experience and believe in your own remembered wellness.

We are living in a time when age-old techniques, like walking and meditation, are being reexplored and tested by modern scientific techniques. And we have much to learn about the mechanisms and the full potential of exercise and meditation for our health, emotional balance, and spiritual clarity.

Yogi Bhajan and Gurucharan Khalsa's book is a wonderful addition to this continuing exploration.

Herbert Benson, M.D., Mind/Body Medical Institute

Dr. Benson is president and founder of the Mind/Body Medical Institute, an associate professor of medicine at Harvard Medical School, and author of *Timeless Healing, The Relaxation Response* and many other books.

Acknowledgments

Developing, teaching, testing, researching, and writing *Breathwalk* was a long and rewarding journey. Along the way, at every step, many people encouraged, supported, and critiqued our efforts. Our sincere thanks and appreciation go to all who helped bring this beautiful technology for the body and mind into accessible programs and into this book.

Thanks to those who took the first steps and walked with us to experience the potentials of the mind, the vital energy of the body, and the dimensions of awareness Breathwalk makes available. Thanks to Dharm Singh Graham for his editing, his aesthetic contributions and for being a research subject; to Jim Brault for teaching and walking with us in the Caribbean; Mark Canaan, who Breathwalked hundreds of miles and who saw its potential; Jagat Joti Singh Khalsa, who was creative and relentless in telling everyone about this program; Hari Kaur Frank, who walked the many miles teaching with us; Dr. John Mack for his wisdom and kindness; Dr. Ed Resnick, whose consistent healing and professional sports therapy experience is second to none; Dr.

Acknowledgments

Candace Royer, department chair in physical education at MIT, who has encouraged us and helped us introduce this to thousands of MIT students and faculty over the last ten years; and Thomas Moore and Hari Kirn who reminded us that the soul of walking is innocence and listening.

We are grateful for the support in time, resources and ideas that allowed us to research the effects of Breathwalk and its components of breathing and meditation. Deep thanks to Dr. Herbert Benson at the Mind/Body Medical Institute who has been gracious, wise and instrumental in our experimental testing. Special thanks to Dr. Ary L. Goldberger at the lab for nonlinear medicine at Beth Israel for his insight and conversations about wellness, and the patterns that rule our health and awareness. Thanks also to the many others who worked to conduct the experiments: Dr. Greg Fricchione, Director of Research in Psychiatry at Brigham and Women's Hospital; Sara Lazar of the Mind/Body Medical Institute; George Bush, M.D. of the Harvard Medical School, Dr. Jeffrey Hausdorff, David Kailton, Amrit Singh Khalsa, Ph.D., of MIT; and the Nuclear Medicine Group at the University of Arizona Medical Center.

Research doesn't happen without generosity and vision by supporters. Our gratitude to: Hari Katie Houlahan, Gessner Geyer of Brainergy, Inc., and Nancy Adams and her husband Dick.

We would like to thank Tony Robbins and his partner Becky Robbins who have encouraged us and given us the opportunity to present Breathwalk to thousands of people through the Life Mastery University. Their unrelenting vision and drive to reach and elevate people's lives matched our desire to give the Breathwalk experience to a wide range of people from many countries.

Acknowledgments

The journey to finish a Breathwalk book was the work of many hands and hearts. From its conception Yogi Bhajan has been the source and inspiration. This is one refreshing sip from a fountain of wisdom he has shared to elevate the lives of each of us. Suzanne Oaks and her assistant Lisa Olney at Broadway Books added exceptional collaborative and editorial skills. Our agent, Joel Fishman of Bedford Bookworks, recognized our potential and used his magic to help find it a place for birth. Many thanks go to Peter Caldwell and Jim Reichert of Business Bookworks who initiated us into the process of creating trade books, edited and critiqued us line by line.

Lastly, nothing would have reached completion without the intelligence, editing, organization, and pure dedication of Gurucharan Kaur Khalsa, C.E.O. of Khalsa Consultants, Inc.

If we have left anyone out it is inadvertent. There have been many people who have taught and helped give Breathwalk to the world. To all our gratitude.

—*Gurucharan Singh Khalsa, Ph.D.*

—*Yogi Bhajan, Ph.D.*

Breathwalk

Introduction

EACH ONE OF US HAS THE VITALITY WITH-
in us to live a healthy, successful life. That vitality comes from body, mind, and spirit
working together. When we experience vitality, we feel alive. We have an inner confidence
that we can embrace our life, accomplish our
goals, and feel our spirit. Vitality resides in the
intricate network of our body, mind, and
spirit. It is our birthright. In this book you
will learn about a powerful, enjoyable way to
vitalize your life: Breathwalk.

Most of us lose touch with that vitality at
times. Life in this day and age has gotten so
busy, time pressured, and complex that it is

difficult to stay in balance. We are all more connected by electronic information networks. Nonetheless we end up with information overload and a longing for more human, heartfelt connections. The many pulls on our time and energy can leave us with inner conflicts and splits we need to harmonize to live a full and vitalized life. In fact, we need some way to stay clear about our purpose and values so we can recognize and act on all the opportunities that come to us.

The vitality we want for a fulfilled life is different from just high energy. Energy has quality as well as quantity. Vitality is when energy comes from all parts of you and acts in harmony, synchronized to the actions you want to take for your purpose. The harmony and synchronized action among all parts matters as much as, if not more than, the strength of any one part. If any single part gets out of tune or out of rhythm with the others, we feel worse and function worse. Internal conflicts literally eat up our energy. The parts in conflict can be the physical organs in our bodies, or they can be subpersonalities within our psyches—one that wants risk versus one that wants security, for instance. Conflicts can arise between any of the parts in our body, mind, and spirit.

Vitality increases as we reduce those inner conflicts and synchronize our many parts to work together. It is the highest quality of energy within us. It sustains us without a letdown. It gives us a sense of control over how we express our energy physically, mentally, and emotionally. Real vitality even touches our spirit and increases our awareness. It is a prime ingredient for a high-quality life.

How Can We Access Our Vitality?

Three keys release that vitality for our use: breath, walking, and attention. All three used together is Breathwalk—the science and art of combining conscious breath and walking into elegant and effective patterns for a healthy, happy, and spirited life. By learning how to consciously breathe and walk, you can elevate your mood, command your energy levels, and shift your mental gears, as you need. Circumstances will cease to drain your energy, hijack your mood, or distract your mind. You can be at peace and rejuvenate, or you can focus your resources to win the day.

Because our vitality comes from our whole being and not just a single part, the best way to reach it is through moderate, systematic exercise that engages to some degree all parts of our body and mind. It's like pushing a swing. One giant thrust can eject an unsuspecting passenger. A little push applied in just the right way, as the swing comes back and reaches its zenith, sends the swing and its delighted passenger steadily and stably higher. That is exactly how Breathwalk builds and releases your inner vitality as it progressively connects you with all the parts of your body, mind, and spirit.

What Is Breathwalk?

Breathwalk is the science of combining specific patterns of breathing synchronized with your walking steps and enhanced with the art of directed, meditative attention. Breathwalk is simple, natural, and effective. Once you know how to choose and do a breathing pattern as you walk, you will have an immediate path to physical and mental fitness.

For most of us, it is as important to have a clear mind and excellent moods as it is to have good physical health and energy. Both are essential to helping us create balance in our lives. When our mind, mood, and energy all work together in a smooth flow, we can effortlessly open up to our spirit and to the wonder that is life.

Breathwalk may seem comfortably familiar to you even though this is your introduction to its practice. That is because it has combined within it many elements that you may have found in other places and in other disciplines.

The emphasis on breathing, and breathing consciously to attain a desired state, has gradually gained widespread recognition, use, and validation. Many training programs for childbirth such as Lamaze use breathing and focused attention to control pain and create deep relaxation. Most forms of martial arts, like karate, judo, win chung, tai chi, and chi gung, use directed breathing to achieve their extraordinary gains in strength and agility. Competitive sports from golf to weight lifting to running have discovered that breath control and using the mind in a meditative way can give an edge to top athletes.

Conscious breathing is also used as a powerful technique in many therapies and approaches to personal growth and transformation. You may have been exposed to some of the breath's possibilities in rebirthing, Grof breathwork, psychoenergetics, Reichian bodywork, or many other related healing disciplines. In the workplace, control of the breath either directly or indirectly with music and evoked feelings has become ubiquitous for reducing the impact of stress. It is taught in many hospital programs for stress control, rehabilitation, and addiction relief.

Meditation has become very popular. One of its primary techniques is to pay attention to the flow of the breath while letting other thoughts lose their command of your consciousness. Buddhist practitioners have shared this technique with millions of Westerners in the last few decades. Practitioners of medical forms of meditation like the relaxation response, taught by Herbert Benson, M.D., use mindfulness in dozens of major medical centers and health care programs around the country. Most universities have some form of meditation in their curricula. Most health clubs and spas also offer classes in meditation.

Another place where you might have heard of or experienced parts of Breathwalk is in a spiritual setting. Many traditions use walking as a meditation to calm the mind, to connect to nature, and for healing. Though walking and Breathwalking are not religious, and do not belong only to one group or culture, they do have strong roots in many spiritual traditions.

Breathwalk is the place where these elements of conscious breathing, walking, and meditation come together. It combines them seamlessly in a very accessible exercise anyone can do. Combining these elements makes the impact greater, the results even more effective. People who Breathwalk often report that it enhances their efforts in other exercise or meditation endeavors.

Breathwalk gives you exercise, personal growth, meditative experience, stress mastery, and a clear mind to feel your spirit more easily. It builds on the base of whatever you have experienced with breath, exercise, and meditation. It takes you just one step further to enhance your practices and add another dimension of choice to your experience.

Proper Breathing Is the Key

Breath is the master key to build and use your vitality. Every cell and part of your body cues off the subtle motions of a breath. Within the rhythms and structure of your breath is coded a language of energy that your nervous system, glands, and mind understand. Breathwalk speaks that code in its simple patterns of breath and movement. You can gather the attention of all parts of your mind and body, change your energy and awareness, and synchronize your parts to work together.

Scientists have shown proper breathing can elevate your mood, create relaxation and shield you from many effects of stress, aid in pain control, and alleviate a wide range of symptoms from headaches to indigestion. After decades of research and an exhaustive review of the literature, Dr. Robert Fried concluded in his 1993 *The Psychology and Physiology of Breathing: In Behavioral Medicine, Clinical Psychology, and Psychiatry* that normal breathing has been overlooked or underemphasized by most physicians and psychiatrists. His studies showed that abnormal breathing patterns, shallow breathing, or hyperventilation is a complication or a causal factor in 50 to 70 percent of medical complaints. By training people in proper breathing, he could alleviate emotional problems, circulatory difficulties, and a range of common complaints.

Dr. Andrew Weil, a strong advocate for self-care and rational use of medicine, sees proper breathing as central to a program of good health and mental balance. In his bestselling 1995 book, *Spontaneous Healing,* Dr. Weil says, "Breathing may be the master function of the body, affecting all others. Restrictions in breathing can be the result of past traumas, both physical and emotional. Most of us have never received instruction about breathing and how to take advantage of it as a harmonizer of mind and body. . . . If breath is the movement of spirit in the body—a central mystery that connects us to all creation—then working with the breath is a form of spiritual practice. It also impacts health and healing, because how we breathe both reflects the state of the nervous system and influences the state of the nervous system. You can learn to regulate heart rate, blood pressure, circulation, and digestion by consciously changing the rhythm and depth of breathing."

Breathwalk trains you in proper breathing so you can achieve all these positive health effects. Then it takes you beyond that. Its special breathing techniques and patterns help you to reach emotional mastery, control your energy level and quality of mind, initiate powerful healing, and accelerate your personal growth.

Proper breathing is first, then conscious breathing, and finally conscious patterned breathing. Combine this with walking and Breathwalk can bring you a wide range of benefits from only a modest effort.

It can help many symptoms and types of problems. We have repeatedly surveyed practitioners of Breathwalk for changes they attribute at least in part to their Breathwalk programs. Although we make no medical claims, Breathwalk in conjunction with other healthy lifestyle choices seems to have a profound healing impact. Most people who reported these effects made other lifestyle changes as well, such as better nutrition, herbal supports, and frequently medical advice or alternative treatments. Breathwalk helped to relieve the following:

Anxiety	*Stress*	*Hypertension*
Depression	*Impulsiveness*	*Emotional trauma*
Back pain	*Obesity*	*Weak immune system*
Fatigue	*Moodiness*	*Poor circulation*
Travel stress	*Inflexibility*	*Addictive impulses*
Feeling overwhelmed	*Low stamina*	*Reduced potency*

The precision and variety in the breath patterns and awakeners in Breathwalk mean we can use its various programs to address and even prevent a surprising range of everyday complaints.

Besides alleviating these kinds of symptoms, the vitality you get from Breathwalk gives you four overarching positive benefits: choice about your energy level, mood control, mental quality, and feeling of connectedness. As you start to get all these benefits from your practice, the sense of spirit and of being part of something greater than one's self increases as well.

The world has changed, and it is going to change more. It is faster, more interconnected, and increasingly complex. Faxes, cell phones, e-mail, television, and the Internet bombard us every day and compete for our attention. The information age brings with it amazing conveniences, but it exacts a toll on our nervous system and on our awareness. To thrive under the impact of this new information ecology that we are creating, we must be able to easily and quickly shift gears. We need to find the calm in the midst of activity. We need to find motivation and focus when we have become scattered. We need to be confident that we can adjust our energy level, direct our mental quality of focus and attention, control our moods, and be open to relationships and collaboration. These are the skills we need to thrive. Breathwalk is a powerful way to get and refine these abilities.

The Four Benefits of Breathwalk

The four main benefits from Breathwalk—increased energy level, mood control, refined mental quality, and feelings of connectedness—have always been important keys to personal growth and effectiveness. They are even more important as we face a future unlike anything we have seen in the past. When you have the resources of these benefits, you have the key to vitality, mental and emotional flexibility, and personal balance as you excel under the pressures of work and changes in your life.

It may seem a little amazing that something as ancient as walking and breathing has emerged as a contemporary solution for balance and vitality. Regardless of how new or futuristic our technology becomes, it still has to interact with our nervous system and mind, which has been shaped from antediluvian roots. We must learn how to regulate our body and mind system to handle our new information environments. Fortunately our nervous and glandular systems, though ancient, are also the most complex, adaptive, and subtle creations that we have found in the universe. If we know how to tap their potentials, we can thrive in this age and the future.

The changes in technology and society that are occurring so rapidly require that we wake up and act consciously. The answer to the challenges of the information age is the rise of an age of awareness where each of us can choose and refine our personal state of mind and energy. Then we can keep a balance within and without. We can act with intelligence and wisdom. Breathwalk brings together ancient wisdom and modern science so we can vitalize ourselves and enjoy each day.

Energy Level

With it we can do everything. Without it the smallest hill becomes a mountain. We begin and end as energy. Think about the beginning of the universe. Suddenly there was light, the big bang flash point, that sent creation out in a wild frenzy of energy, elements, and potential awareness. We still contain the seeds of that primal light energy and all the complexity of the elements. Everything we do of any significance still depends on our ability to tap and regulate energy. We use chemical energy for metabolism, and mechanical energy for movement and action. Electrical energy connects all our cells and gives us the miracles of perception and awareness in our nervous system. And, in a very subtle form, we radiate light and energy as an aura that expresses our spirit. Every day feels like a success when we generate enough energy to sustain our actions and our radiance. Breathwalk is one of the best energy generators that we've come across. When you need to adjust your energy lower to relax or higher to perform, take a Breathwalk.

Mood Control

Moods are important because they form the background, the canvas, on which our thoughts shape the experience of our lives. Our mood affects what memories we can reach, the stream of thoughts we tune in to, and how we use our energy levels. Mood, thought, and energy relate in a complex dance within each one of us.

To be alive is to have rhythms and to have emotional ups and downs. We cannot always be up, living life in the emotional stratosphere. We can accept, and even value, mild mood downswings. They can add depth to our feelings and to our empathy for other people.

When moods get stuck so they are not appropriate for what we want to do or express, then we have a problem. Moods are a bit like an emotional default, an automatic emotional base. For times in history when everything changed slowly, this worked great. Now we live in a time that requires much more emotional fluidity. We get stuck more often if we don't do something to consciously change.

The result is a disturbing trend and statistic. Cases of depression have risen twentyfold in the twentieth century. Even with all our new drugs, as a group we suffer from increasing mood distress—anxiety, depression, hyperactive distraction, and fatigue. We need ways to take charge of our moods and smoothly align them to our purposes. Mood states can be altered, shifted from their negative to their positive form just as a photographic negative can yield a positive print.

We have found that specific Breathwalk patterns can actually shift the mood state in specific ways: from anxious to calm; from depressed to hopeful; and from worried to confident. These shifts originate in the interaction of exercise and the complex neurochemistry of the body. The right physical movements synchronized with the breath and with some mental sounds to counter negative internal self-talk change moods effectively. The variety of Breathwalk patterns this book offers will give you choice and control over your ordinary moods and alleviate many forms of moderate depression.

Mental Quality

Have you ever noticed that when your energy level falls, you have trouble thinking clearly? Energize the nervous system and the clarity of your mind increases. Breathwalk's effects upon mental clarity and focus only begin with energy. Have competing thoughts and desires ever besieged you? The conflicting thoughts can keep you from focusing effectively. You lose track of what is important and stray from your real purpose. We all have such scattered moments, but we can choose to shift from scattered to focused and be the director of our mind. We can consciously train our minds to become obedient servants, not capricious masters, of our will. Specific patterns of rhythm, action, and thought built right into Breathwalk can help you achieve that mastery over your own mind. Some Breathwalkers describe the change in their mind as going from fog to a clear sky. Others say it is like going from black and white to color or from a flat two-dimensional image to a full three-dimensional one.

Connectedness

This is a powerful benefit that is increasingly important to our personal balance and effectiveness. Under pressure and change it is natural to withdraw. We contract, hide under the covers, and restrict our contact and connections with others. When we are healthy in body and mind, we react differently. We stay open and even feel vast and connected to people, to life and nature, and to ourselves.

The dictionary defines "connectedness" as 1) joined together; 2) associated or related; or 3) intelligently ordered. That is a good definition of this benefit. When you breathe vitality into your body, mind, and spirit with a Breathwalk, it opens your senses and frees your feelings. You can feel the larger whole that you are part of as well as your individual part. Nature and the flow of your life seem to have an intelligent order. You can perceive how things are connected to each other and make better choices about how to get from one point to another. You can naturally feel your spirit. You can Breathwalk alone and know you are not alone—know that you have connections.

Breathwalk can improve your connectedness in relationships, even intimate relationships. It shifts your energy and mood, but it is also by nature a relational exercise. You can do it with a partner. You and your partner can move in the same pattern. You can leave behind your old stuck states as you breathe new energy into your feelings. You can alternate between a stroll with conversation and a Breathwalk pattern that opens your heart and mind. At the end of a Breathwalk the gap between your minds and hearts is narrowed. You are connected and will find it easier to communicate.

The Spiritual Benefits of Breathwalk

We rarely ask people to do Breathwalk for a spiritual experience. Such things flow from private and intimate motivations, and the spirit is spontaneous. Many people, however, do report deep changes from Breathwalking—they tell us of feeling connected to their spirit vividly for the first time. They cease feeling alone and sense that people who love them have become a part of them. They can feel each other and respond without effort. They may even share the same thoughts at the same time. That delicious sense of relatedness extends to work, to all the people they encounter, and to nature. Spirit has no limit, and neither does our connection with it.

Spirit is something we all have. It's spoken about in a thousand ways. It doesn't require any particular belief, though it can enliven our experience of our beliefs. It does require an engagement. It thrives when we invite it in and discover its dimensions within us and our lives. It is not something that can be forced or chased and captured. It is as spectacular as a splendiferous sunrise and as hidden as the stars in midday light. To radiate spirit and the deep vitality it bestows takes awareness, innocence, and integrity. With those qualities in us we sparkle until the spirit picks us up.

Breathwalking with the flow of a conscious breath as you meditate is a way to offer that invitation to the spirit. It has been used for as long as people have lived. Perhaps breath is a natural front door into the house of spirit. We live only because of the gentle pulse of our breath. Many traditions sense that spirit in the body is expressed by breath. So as we walk and consciously breathe, we are inviting in the spirit and giving a place to converse with our soul. The hearth in such a house is awareness. The food we share with our subtle guest is our elevated words infused with a radiant and focused mind.

We deeply need to take time for our spirit. It is not a gimmick or something that our minds can command. It shows up with equal urgency in our times of brightness and in our periods of darkness. Embracing our spirit is something our modern culture has marginalized, but that embrace is the very balance that we need to be vital and content as we progress into a globalized and interconnected world.

Take a look at the case of Linda. Linda came down with cancer—non-Hodgkin's lymphoma. The prognosis was not good. She had been practicing the techniques of meditation, healing massage, and Breathwalk, but when we first saw Linda after her diagnosis her face was thunderstruck with grief. We talked for a long time. Then she went for a long Breathwalk through the local woods by a beautiful reservoir. When she returned her face was bright. She told us that she had walked and breathed, she had watched all the activity of the birds and animals, and she was seized with an amazing feeling. All of a sudden she felt strongly that this was her chance to change her life! This was the moment when she could choose to be true to herself and act on her real priorities. The following week, Linda showed me a notebook that listed all of the changes she had already made. I asked her what she would feel if the treatments failed. Her reply was simple. "Live or die, I will have changed and woken up." Linda had gotten in touch with her invincible spirit and vitality and inspired us all.

In his 1992 *Care of the Soul: A Guide for Cultivating Depth and Sacredness in Everyday Life*, Thomas Moore identified the importance of giving time to the soul this way: "The great malady of the 20th century implicated in all of our troubles and affecting us individually and socially is 'loss of soul.' When soul is neglected, it doesn't go away; it appears symptomatically in obsessions, addictions, violence and loss of meaning . . . it is impossible to define the soul." His thoughtful observations show that the spirit appears in many forms but always as a force that seems to connect us more firmly to life and to our vitality to live it.

When the spirit becomes awakened within us, we find our bodies newly energized and our minds hosting a new awareness. The spirit quickens qualities within us that we often are surprised we possess. When we experience the opening of the spirit, it renews and refreshes like soft, falling rain. The body becomes more sensitive to everything around us. Life becomes magnetized with a new ability to read the meaning of things. We stop judging and start serving. We cease useless rationalizations and commit to act.

The spirit is tangible. It is not hidden. We can feel it and see it. It even emits a glow and puts lightness into our steps as we walk.

How We Developed the Breathwalk Program

I, Gurucharan, met Yogi Bhajan in 1969 at a lecture he was giving at the Claremont Colleges. He was a master yogi and a spiritual teacher who had recently arrived from India. I was an American-born doctoral student in mathematics. It was East meets West, a perfect combination. Yogi Bhajan had come to openly share the wisdom of the ages that until then had been passed on only orally within guarded and secret traditions. He did this with a rare combination of personal depth, intuition, practicality, and integrity. He was a yogi in the truest sense of the word. My urge was to learn everything he knew and then to hold it up to the rigorous light of scientific analysis. I was a scientist. Since that first meeting I have never stopped learning from Yogi Bhajan's wisdom. Over the last thirty years we have worked together

to teach hundreds of thousands of people how to live a fulfilled life—healthy, happy, and holy.

We have both worked in social programs such as juve-
nile diversion, drug rehabilitation, and prisons. Since ob-
taining doctorates in psychology, each of us has maintained
separate individual and family counseling practices allowing us to coach people from every walk of life, including
business executives, athletes, artists, and spiritual seekers of
all kinds.

One of our shared goals is to make available to everyone the most effective and practical techniques for personal
growth and healing based on the combination of ancient
yogic wisdom and modern science. From the beginning we
have taught the positive impact of exercise, breath, and
meditation. We have created practical programs everyone
can use to make their lives a little better. Breathwalk is one
such program. We have used it in a wide variety of applica-
tions: to end addictions, to help young students deal with
their feelings, in therapeutic settings for groups and individuals, with couples who want to create stronger relationships, and in many other settings.

The results of teaching Breathwalk have always been
positive and often astounding. We were able to describe the
effects of Breathwalking from anecdotal reports and personal experience. We understood the Eastern philosophy
behind the energetic changes induced by the application of
breath and meditation, but we wanted to also understand
the effects based on modern physiology and scientific research. So, to substantiate the effects of combining breath,
walking, and meditation, we initiated surveys on moods,
made recordings of physiological rhythms, and even monitored the brain with PET scans and MRIs to see how the
brain changed from these breathing and walking patterns.

Breathwalk

We are excited to share the results of this research along with these techniques in this book.

The use of exercise, conscious breathing, and meditation has broadened our lives and given us the vitality to serve people in every part of the world. It has given us a way to help people transform themselves and live to their full potential.

We have been inspired to create this book by the many people who have shared their stories of life-changing transformation achieved through Breathwalking. The Jazzman is one such true story.

The Jazzman

Dave composes music—jazz rhythms—and teaches at the Berklee School of Music in Boston. Some years ago his music grew in popularity, until he found himself in demand as a world-class performer as well as a teacher. He was invited to perform in Europe, South America, Africa, and all over the United States. Audiences were hungry for his stimulating, spontaneous talent. The safe, predictable world of the classroom vaporized, and he found himself, as many of us would, getting anxious. Sweat came to his brow, and his mind became distracted and agitated. His confidence lagged.

We had met a few years earlier through his wife, who attends the Thursday night class in Cambridge. Dave was skeptical of meditation, and it was hard for him to believe walking could be of any real help in handling feelings as intense as his. But after some encouragement from his wife, he decided he couldn't see any downside to just trying it out.

Together Dave and I worked out a simple Breathwalk

program to counter his anxiety and panic attacks. We also chose Breathwalk programs to build up the energy and power of his personal projection—his stage presence. He took on the Breathwalk with dedicated regularity. His initial skepticism disappeared within a week of practice. Then he was filled with questions and wanted to learn all the ways he could use it. In a matter of a few months he mastered his anxiety.

We both often walk along the Charles River in Boston between MIT and the Berklee School of Music. Our paths crossed on the Massachusetts Avenue Bridge. I asked him, "Are you performing tonight or listening to someone else's concert?"

He said, "Just listening. But I don't have any more trouble with my anxiety. I'm steady as a rock. Audiences, big or small, don't bother me. That 4/4 Breathwalk rhythm and a fifteen-minute walk knocks the edge off anything that starts up. Now my mind just goes to jazz and all jazz, no more mental spinning."

We kept walking together and pretty soon found ourselves picking up speed and doing the 4/4 breathing rhythm together. We synchronized it to our walking pace. When we slowed to a regular walk he continued his story. "I started Breathwalk to cope with my anxiety. Now I use it if I need a little extra energy, or at the end of a late night set when my mind keeps working instead of letting me sleep. When I first started, I was willing to try anything. I thought it would be a lot of effort, but it wasn't. It was easy and now it's fun, and I don't think much about it—I just do it. It's like a good beat that lets me catch the rhythm of my day." We parted with a smile.

It's the many stories and successes like the Jazzman's that proved to us the power and benefits of Breathwalk. It was from the many comments people shared with us about the personal benefits of Breathwalk that we recognized the four main benefits we discussed before.

This book is intended for people who have never exercised regularly but who want to start. It is also for those with a great exercise or meditation practice who want to increase their range and depth of experience. Our experience is that as you learn the programs that relate to your goals, Breathwalk will support and expand your life.

The book takes you step by step to full confidence in exactly how to do Breathwalk. We start with the benefits to make you aware of the possibilities and to motivate you to try it. Once you try Breathwalk the experience will speak for itself. Then in two chapters we cover the basics of breathing. We look at normal complete breathing, then at special breaths and patterns that we use in Breathwalk. Chapter 4 takes you for a walk. It is an experiential description of a Breathwalk from beginning to end. It gives you the big picture in a few pages. The next five chapters describe each of the five steps of Breathwalk in detail: awaken, align, vitalize, balance, and integrate. We cover the ideas behind each step as well as how to do them. In the next chapter we describe the use of sounds with your programs. Then in one chapter we discuss the results of our research on the impact of Breathwalk. We conclude with spirit and a little history of how people have used walking to deepen themselves and their experience of life. The last section of the book consists of a guide. It explains each program and gives instructions for how to do the awakener exercises and the patterns—everything you need to do to begin a practice and to open your world with Breathwalk.

The Breathwalk Time Bonus

The programs are designed so you can slip them into a busy life no matter how packed your schedule may be. When you begin Breathwalk, you immediately earn a bonus, a time bonus. You gain back the time you invest. This is as important to many people as all the other benefits. They feel time is the greatest block to acting on what they already know will give them vitality and happiness. Breathwalk is a practice that gives you an edge over time.

Some of the hardest choices we make in our modern lives revolve around time: How much of it do we give to each competing activity in life? We sometimes feel that we just cannot give up the sort of time that any regular exercise takes. After all, the total time for a great Breathwalk can easily be one-half to three-quarters of an hour. If you start to think, This is going to be a lot of time out of my day; I'm not sure I can spare that much time, just consider this: When you take the time to Breathwalk, you get the time back plus interest through the rest of the day. You can actually use Breathwalk as a *time creator.*

How can this be true? How can giving a half hour to an hour or so out of a day to Breathwalk create more time for you? There is a simple explanation. You live on human biological time, not on the mechanical time of a clock. Our human time is far richer than clock time. We gain more human time when we get more done in the same tick of the clock. We can pack more experience into the same moment. We can use our intuition to sense the flow of things and leverage each of our efforts with an effortless synchronization of events. Breathwalk gives you heightened focus and intuitive powers that remain with you throughout the day. You keep functioning at 80 to 100 percent of your top performance rather than slumping and limping along at 25 percent for periods during the day.

Even a short Breathwalk—a ten- to fifteen-minute Breathwalk exercise at work—can boost you right back to full vitality and top performance. You will find that you become far more productive whatever your pursuit. Operating with invincible vitality and its increased awareness, you will find that you have actually gained back more useful time than you gave up doing Breathwalk in the first place.

There is one more facet to this time bonus. Breathwalk practitioners consistently report an increase in "synchronicity"—the meaningful coincidence that seems like luck but accomplishes your key purpose as if the universe gave you a helping hand. Call it enhanced intuitive effectiveness or the angel factor; it gets you from where you are to where you want to go in no time at all.

With Breathwalk the time you expend gives you time for the rest of your life. Breathwalk does not compete for time from other activities. It creates time to support what is important in your life.

Now that you know the background of how we created Breathwalk, what it is, and some of its benefits, you are ready to begin. Breathwalk is the science and art of consciously combining breath and walking, to vitalize your body, mind, and spirit. The result is increased health, pleasure in life, and clarity in your mind. We hope this introduction has piqued your curiosity and interest. This is just the beginning. It's a wonderful journey we have both walked and that we welcome you to explore.

1 Improving Energy, Mood, Mind, and Connectedness

BREATHWALK PROGRAMS CAN VITALIZE YOUR body, mind, and spirit. That special vitality you get from a Breathwalk gives you four main benefits—increased energy levels, mood control, refined mental quality, and feelings of connectedness. Those benefits are like states in America. Each state has its own character, culture, and ways of behaving. Each benefit has its own characteristics and behaviors. Think about it: to really enjoy a visit to a state, you need to look a little more closely at the travel guide in order to see the cities and the special features in the environment that you want to experience. Consider this chapter a closer look at the territory of each benefit. We will identify certain noteworthy features of its terrain, giving you the information you need to design an exploration that will give you the kind of experience you want.

Part of the beauty of Breathwalk is that it gives you a wide spectrum of choices. It is rich with variety, even though its foundation, walking and breathing, is simple. Once you know which pattern of exercise and breathing to do, you can target specific shifts in your energy levels, your mood, and your awareness and achieve amazing results.

In this chapter we will take you through each of the types of Breathwalk benefits. You might be pleasantly surprised to find so many choices within each benefit. After all, Breathwalk is not just exercise. It is exercise plus a meditative mind. Add to that specific patterns of breath and you can design your walking experience with as much nuance as you like.

A Breathwalk can be divided into five steps that flow from one to the other in each walk. These steps are awaken, align, vitalize, balance, and connect. Each Breathwalk offers you so many choices because the different exercises, breathing patterns, and ways of using your mind's attention can be combined in a variety of ways in every walk. We will go through each of these five Breathwalk steps in detail in later chapters, but first let's talk in more detail about the four main benefits of the Breathwalk program.

Benefit 1. Increased Energy Levels

Our personal energy level affects our lives in multifaceted ways. Energy determines our capacity for elegant action in the world. Energy bounds the intensity with which we can express ourselves. It determines, for instance, our ability to speak powerfully—with animation and impact. When our energy level is optimal, we become aroused and alerted to the world around us. Then, with a profound reciprocity, nature seems alerted to and connected to us. We experience energy as vigor and stamina—the physical and mental strength that we can sustain and bring to bear upon any problem.

We all feel our energy in its potential and active forms. We sense our reserves as well as our immediate energy and use our assessment of both to determine which challenges we will take on and which we will decline. And one of our greatest sources for reserve energy is our spirit. Whether we recognize it or not, when we reach deeply within ourselves and tap into our spirit, that spirit gives us stamina, grit, scope, and energy that works regardless of everything happening around us.

Even though our energy level has multiple areas of expression and corresponding sources, most of us form habits and consistently draw our energy from a few favored yet unhealthy sources. Instead of drawing on the body-mind-spirit as a whole, we grab on to seemingly immediate solutions like food, drugs, emotional dramas, or excitement. But our design is subtler than that. Our sources are more diverse. We need to think more holistically about our energy level and its sources, for as we'll explain further in a moment, quick fixes like food and drugs actually take away more energy than they provide. Breath, on the other hand, works as an energy source. It is one we don't use enough. Huge reserves of energy lie buried in our musculature and in our glands, ready to be tapped and used—by mastering our own breathing.

You see, the nervous system can actually contain and release energy. The part of your nervous system called the autonomic system can be developed in the same way that a muscle can be toned or shaped. And the energy stored or released in that system is directly affected by breathing, exercise, and your entire attitude. Your emotions, and all the electrical and chemical processes that change with them, are sources for energy. Awareness itself is also a great source of energy, for your state of awareness directly changes the pattern of your brain activity. Good, healthy nutrition and conscious eating is another source of energy and healing. Our ideal is to be vitalized by all these sources. We want to align our habits and activities to sources of energy that deliver us in the present and sustain us for the future.

But without some training and conscious introspection, most of us do not use all of these sources. Instead, once we sense our energy is running low, we let our search for more energy get directed by unconscious habits and emergency reflexes. We grasp whatever seems closest and takes the least attention or effort. Surrounded by junk food and instant everything, we often make poor choices and end up *losing* energy instead of gaining it. A drink or two to relax at the end of the day seems reasonable, but for many people it leads to depression, reckless driving, and emotional withdrawal. Not knowing how to tap our core energy, some of us rely on stirring up an emotional storm within ourselves. The resulting emotional outburst releases energy but, like a bad storm, devastates everything in its path—a short-term gain, but an enduring loss that actually depletes our energy. In order to get and stay vitalized and healthy for the long run, however, we need to cultivate effective energy regeneration strategies. Like a flowing stream, we need constant renewal to live well.

What good energizing strategies should we adopt, then? Over the years we have found that exercise is one of the best. For while we do get a temporary energy shift from certain outside sources like drugs or overeating, these short-term gains come at a high long-term cost, such as temporary depression, illness and allergies, or loss of focus and anxiety. Exercise has none of these downsides. It is a great and consistent energy generator. You may have noticed you feel much more energized after even moderate exercise. In fact, a recent study reported in the January 27, 1999, issue of the *Journal of the American Medical Association* showed that moderate increases in walking even done in small amounts during the normal workday yield great benefits in energy and cardiovascular health. Those people who learned to use walking during the day maintained the gains more than those engaging in more structured workouts in gyms. And they didn't even have to make drastic changes in their lives. These people did things like taking longer walks on the way to office meetings, walking around airports instead of sitting while waiting for a plane, walking around a soccer field at children's games, and walking together socially.

The Breathwalk program is a great way to get all those benefits and more. As you'll see, exercise, breath, and awareness combine for explosive, sustainable gains in your energy level. Listen to the difference it made in the life of Julie, a chiropractor and mother in Vermont who sent us this e-mail after practicing Breathwalk for a year. "I used to come home with no energy for my children. I even considered starting a new business since I value my family and my peace so much. Breathwalk has recharged me. It has changed my life! I now have enough energy when I do a Breathwalk at the end of the workday that I can really be present with my children. I have no urge to withdraw, and I don't feel like yelling. This is a lifesaver."

Most of us have had the experience of a sudden,

unexpected surge in energy when presented with a new opportunity or pleasant temptation. For instance, we may return home from work feeling exhausted—until a friend calls up and suggests playing a demanding athletic game or going somewhere exciting. Then we perk right up. Novelty itself calls up new possibilities and old associations to produce immediate energy, but unlike the Breathwalk program, it is not a lasting energy.

We can gain energy by losing weight when we are overweight. We can also boost energy by gaining weight when we are under our ideal. Breathwalk can work as a highly effective program to adjust your weight up or down. It optimizes the available energy in body, mind, and emotions. Once this is balanced, you instinctively reshape your weight.

We can call on our energy in different forms and with different qualities. Three qualities of energy are familiar and practical to most people. When we build our vitality, we build on all three. One is energy for immediate quick action. It is short-lived and needs constant replenishment from your activity or from your reserves. A second is like a reservoir. It is energy on hand in reserve and can be tapped gradually in large amounts or more quickly in small amounts. It is in your glands, fat, nerve, and muscle and helps keep away illness and support daily functions. A third form of energy is distributed and held in patterns of tension and emotion. We can release, gather, and redirect this energy, interrupt automatic patterns that stored it for some purpose, and use it consciously for what is most important. Together these three forms of energy give you superior performance and a life sparkling with vitality.

The best approach to build and maintain these three forms of your energy is to form helpful habits—habits that give you natural energy maintenance each day. The correct Breathwalk patterns will do precisely this. Done daily, or at least five times weekly, these exercise patterns will assure that you always possess the energy you want. There are Breathwalks that build each of these three energy sources in you.

Our most potent forms of energy come not from outside ourselves, but from within. Our bodies and our minds hold energy in their patterns of attention and tension. When we draw upon our nervous system, mind, and spirit, we concentrate or release energy without side effects and reactions. Vigor and vitality come when the use of all your sources of energy are aligned with the action you want to take or the state you want to be in. Drawing upon all your healthy inner and outer sources in a balanced manner multiplies the effect obtained from only one or two of these sources. We have found that the best way to maximize your vital energy is to eat nutritiously (and judiciously), forgo drug and alcohol use, exercise moderately, embrace new and novel opportunities in life, and engage in effective breathing and meditative exercises like Breathwalk.

Benefit 2. Mood Control

Imagine how life feels when we have a positive, flexible mood. Life flows steadily like a great river traversing the open plains, and our thoughts and actions align with its movements effortlessly. Life appears vibrant—pulsating, pushing, enticing, and caressing us—and yet calm at the very center. Life fills full with reasons for living. It needs nothing else for motivation and enables our innate, spiritual disposition to express what we care about most and see it reach a healthy fruition. When our mood and mind come together in this way, we live truly happy, healthful, and holy lives.

An elevated, positive mood is a powerful, galvanizing asset for living a vitalized life. But what can we do when our mood flips from positive to negative? For in this day and age, having your life flow calmly like a deep, powerful river is increasingly rare. The accelerated pace of daily living and the overbearing burdens of the volume of information that is thrust upon us make it so. Stress and anxiety shift inward from the world around us and imprint themselves onto our bodies. Sometimes that tension builds into a negative, oppressive mood. It descends heavily like a thick fog over our relationships and dreams and shatters any harmony we might have among our moods, thoughts, and efforts. Or that tension simply intensifies until it gradually manifests itself as an illness or chronic fatigue.

Stress and pressure can stimulate us in small doses. When it comes along with a well-focused effort and goal like training for a marathon, it can actually have a positive effect. But pressure that comes all the time, from every quarter, is like a river full of angry rapids and treacherous shallows running onward to crushing falls. Our moods respond with their own turbulence, furtive feelings, and reactions filled with misjudgments, and instead of being able to flow smoothly with the river of life, we thrash out or merely drift. Motivation becomes distant, and a chilling depression can settle in. Our emotions and moods go from being helpful friends to becoming our worst pitfall.

But moods in all their vicissitudes can be mastered. In fact, mood control is not only possible but readily and simply available to us. And when we achieve mood mastery, our emotions jump in line and prepare us to act effectively and with power. They gather our thoughts, set our inner energy level, and alert needed areas in our body and mind. With emotional readiness and action synchronized to work together, we can easily jump into the flow and rhythm of life—no matter what the turbulence or pace. With total vitality we can engage the challenges of the day and make it look easy. We can find our balance and feel the profound presence of our spirit. We can reach a profound confidence and contentment when we experience a healthy relation to the flow of our feelings, thoughts, and actions.

It does not have to take years of treatment by a professional therapist or doctor to achieve significant choice and control over the ups and downs of our moods, although counseling and professional assessment are always prudent and can certainly help, especially if the moods are extreme. On our own, however, we can do a lot to affect our moods. One of the largest impacts we can make comes through physical exercise, and especially breathing with moderate walking. Moods have a physical basis in our body chemistry. This means that psychology can follow physiology just as easily as the other way around. The breathing patterns in Breathwalk can send a kind of code, a set of instructions, that can activate areas of our brain like the hypothalamus to mobilize our nerves and hormones—immediately altering our mood state.

Moods that are out of control are costly to us as individuals and as a society. One estimate of the economic impact as reported in *The New York Times* was over $43 billion annually in 1995. Of that, $23 billion was due to lost productivity. And those figures have gone up every year. Yet there is certainly hope. The 1996 Surgeon General's Report, *Physical Activity and Health,* stated that there is substantial research to support the claim that moderate exercise like walking provides significant relief for depression, anxiety, and other mood problems. In fact, the benefits begin on the very first session of exercise. Furthermore, this natural approach supports and accelerates counseling and drug approaches. So we can shift the physiological state in our bodies and the attention in our mind to direct and set our psychological experience.

Choosing to have control over your moods has a real, down-to-earth basis to it. Your breath, posture, and rhythm allow you to change your mood. Even a dark thought loses its grip on the mind with a proper change in breathing and attention. Knowing that you have a choice about how you're feeling also lets you learn from your mood. Sometimes moods are filled with messages about how we need to change. When we can feel them and have a choice to alleviate them, it is easier to understand what it is about them that is important.

Michael is a computer security specialist for a major New York financial firm. He has had bouts with depression and compulsiveness for many years and takes medications to alleviate them. But Michael just wasn't happy with the feeling of dependency on drugs; he wanted to have more choices available to him. In coordination with his therapist, Michael decided to begin a regular program of Breathwalks aimed at his particular moods. His comment after a few months was, "I feel bigger than my moods. It's like a space opened up. Instead of being small and pressed into a corner, I can move. My therapist lowered my medication by half. I can do the walk every day, even in the building I work at. Ten minutes here and there smooth me right out. I have also begun to understand how I need to handle conflicts in my life differently. I guess I already knew that, but I realized it clearly during one of the Innerwalks at the end of the Hawk Breathwalk with the 8/4 breath that you showed me." It has been two years now since Michael made that comment, and he has been able to maintain the benefits and increase his sense of choice for the entire period.

Knowing how to change your moods and trusting in that is exhilarating. Smoothly switching moods is like using paddles to go from fast-moving to slower-moving currents in a river. We can play in the churning eddies and backwashes or enter still, dark waters that bring us calm. The pull of the current is welcome because you are ready for whatever comes.

Later in this book we'll show you the Breathwalks to accomplish the specific mood shifts we will look at now. Each of these shifts is useful and valuable to having your moods support and vitalize your life.

There are four common mood upsets that we have all come across: anxiety, depression, irritated distraction, and a lack of motivation. We can shift each of these to a more positive state with the proper patterns of Breathwalk. Let's look closely at what each shift is like.

Four Types of Mood Shifts

SIMPLE ANXIETY SHIFTED TO INNER CALM. The most common mood upset appears as simple anxiety. We worry excessively. We fix our minds upon unimportant details, and then we churn and grind away on them. Yet we never seem to get them ground down to nothing. We rush to clean out our closets when we should finish a job or make the deadline for our taxes. As a nation, we spend many billions of dollars for tranquilizing drugs, yet we remain overwrought.

Breathwalk

Sometimes it helps just to stand back and withdraw from things for a while. To get some distance from the troublesome feelings, we need to change the patterns of tension in our body with a burst of physical activity. Anxiety can be held and rutted into our body by unconscious breathing patterns and muscular rigidity. Breathwalk can work out all that tension and redirect our attention so that we can let go of our own anxious thoughts and feelings.

DEPRESSED SHIFTED TO CLEAR AND CONNECTED. In normal depressions our energy level plummets and we feel disconnected from the things that matter to us. We often lose our vision of the future. We surround ourselves with negative thoughts that seem to counter, like a dead weight, any action we desire to take. The ability to change this mood quickly is essential in this age of rapid changes and dislocations.

DISTRACTED, BUSY, AND HYPERACTIVE SHIFTED TO RECEPTIVE AND INTIMATE. Keeping a good balance between the workplace and home is important to most of us. Often we can have trouble switching our mood states between the two—leaving the driven, purposeful pace at work to become receptive to new things in our home lives. Yet that mood switch after work holds one of the keys to keeping the relationships we value in good order. If you don't recenter quickly, it's like having an intimate dinner while one of you reads the newspaper or the stock quotes—physical presence, but a great emotional divide. There are several Breathwalk exercises that have saved a lot of relationships over the years and are great to do with partners at the end of the day.

DOUBTFUL AND LETHARGIC SHIFTED TO MOTIVATED AND READY. Frequently we have to pull ourselves together to meet a particularly demanding situation, such as speaking to a large group. We may need to take charge of a meeting, or of our family and children, but feel unsure about being able to do it. We need to get motivated, get focused, and take the leap. At such times we can call upon the inner resources we possess. This shift is great for many business situations as well as for just getting out of bed to go enjoy the day on that Sunday we finally have for ourselves.

For each of these shifts we'll give you the specific Breathwalk patterns to help. The details are in the guide at the back of this book.

Benefit 3. Refined Mental Quality

Conquer your mind, and you conquer the world. Conquer the mind, and challenge becomes opportunity, failure becomes learning, and every success brings gratitude and balance. Almost unlimited power resides within us, in our own minds. We need only release it. Everything depends upon the relationship we have with our own minds.

One place where we can easily see the impact of our relationship with our minds is in the placebo effect. This is an effect that results from a patient's expectation, belief, or mind-set about a treatment and the doctor or healer giving the treatment. In many medical experiments subjects are given an "active" drug or treatment and a control that is "inactive." So to treat depression, for example, one group is given a real antidepressant and the other is given water, sugar, or some other neutral substance. In *The Placebo Effect:*

An Interdisciplinary Exploration, published by Harvard University Press in 1999, the contributors showed clear evidence that the placebo acted as well as an active drug or other treatment in 40–65 percent of the cases depending on the particular experiment.

A positive mind that can focus on a clear expectation is amazingly powerful. There are many debates about the exact mechanisms, but one thing is for sure: It all depends on the state of your mind and its focus. On October 13, 1998, *The New York Times* reported that placebos "are about 55 to 60 percent as effective as most active medications like aspirin and codeine for controlling pain." Of more interest to us is the conclusion in the same article that healing is triggered by the state of our mind. "Can a thought or belief produce a chemical cascade that leads to healing and wellness? Researchers studying placebos think the answer is yes. . . . Using new techniques of brain imagery, they are uncovering a host of biological mechanisms that can turn a thought, belief or desire into an agent of change in cells, tissues and organs." A single positive thought clearly held can release a cascade of curative effects throughout our entire beings. Breathwalk gives you a way to immediately and directly affect your mind and its flow of thoughts. That is a great power and a marvelous benefit.

We can relate to our own minds in one of two ways: We have either a conscious relationship with our minds or an unconscious relationship. When our relationships with our own minds reach a conscious level, our minds become our best servants. So long as the relationship remains unconscious, however, our minds will remain our worst masters. Then we must act at the whim of the thousands of thoughts our minds produce each moment. Uncontrolled, the mind becomes a prolific random thought generator.

Those thoughts pound and scatter us like a hammer making shards out of glass.

But we *can* make our minds conscious allies. The power of a conscious relationship to our own mind and awareness has been documented and explained by Harvard researcher Ellen J. Langer in her 1997 book, *The Power of Mindful Learning*. Dr. Langer sums up the results of dozens of studies by concluding, "A mindful approach to any activity has three characteristics: the continuous creation of new categories; openness to new information; and an implicit awareness of more than one perspective." The Breathwalk program uses mindful attention during walking, and as a result, our mind will be primed for learning, creativity, and getting out of old ruts of thinking and feeling.

We can begin to consciously direct and develop the mind with the resources that we've already identified—energy and mood. Energy is the beginning: Energize the nervous system, and the power of the mind increases. Synchronize mind and mood, and we team up our intellect and our feelings to become intelligent in our actions. With energy and an elevated mood, we have kindled the flame and power of our minds. Now add to that the benefits of a clear and conscious mind, and create a powerful inner light—a vitalized mind.

The same information overload that affects our energy and mood also affects how well we perceive information and how our mind makes decisions. Just imagine going to a meeting at work or to a party with friends at night. Now imagine going with severe jet lag or a lack of sleep. Immediately our minds seek a strategy to cope with all the stimulation. Withdraw to a corner. Take extra drugs. Pick a few well-known people and anchor to them like the moon to the earth. We may look as though we are present, but mentally we are only partly there. Our decisions become as fuzzy as our perceptions. To defend against the stress, our minds can just lock up, and as a result we lose focus. We begin to define the problems facing us in the wrong way and go in circles, looking for solutions to the wrong problems. This was the situation facing a woman named Marielle, but listen to how she was able to use a specific Breathwalk to change all that.

Marielle is an air traffic controller in Canada. After several years on the job she decided she had to take a stress leave. She felt she had to leave her job because it was destroying her health, and she felt her judgment was getting fuzzy under the constant pressure. We talked and decided she would learn and practice Breathwalk during her sabbatical as she reexamined her choices. After three months she wrote, "My feet are on the ground. I have my old energy back. But it's more than that. I have a center. And from that center I can see that I love doing this and I can do it well. I need to take care of myself. Keep my balance. Just 'brassing' through won't work, and there was never any reason it should. Breathwalk is amazing. An hour seems like a short walk now. At the end of every walk my eyes seem to get so clear that it's like looking for the first time and catching all of the details I usually miss. And my mind is pure crystal. Clear. Strong. Thank you." Not long after receiving Marielle's note, we heard that she had resumed her job. She's still there today.

There are four qualities of the mind that enhance its power and prevent the problems of stress and overload. If we maintain and enhance these four qualities in combination with a good energy level and a mood appropriate to our challenges, we have the most direct approach for vitalized living. Use the Breathwalk program to boost these four qualities of the mind and to simultaneously form a conscious relationship to the mind. By using specific exercises, we can sweep out all the old cobwebs from our minds, welcome new information and feelings, and take charge of our minds' faculties for clear, intuitive, focused, and creative thought.

Four Qualities of Mind

1. MENTAL CLARITY. With mental clarity, all our senses open and become receptive to information, both inner and outer. The confusion that comes from inner conflict is a great enemy of clarity. When we argue between parts of ourselves, or debate between the past and the future, we cloud our clarity and decrease our ability to apply the mind with singular integrity. Clarity for problems in the world starts with clarity within ourselves. With Breathwalk we increase our clarity when we raise our energy, become consciously conscious, and control our inner dialogue.

2. INTUITION. Everyone has the potential for good intuition. It is built into the very structure of the mind and is supported by the use of the whole brain. These properties define the intuitive power of the mind: see beyond the surface of things, to attend to things not seen well by our rational mind alone, to use all of the implicit as well as explicit learning available to us, and to recognize and know something with certainty beyond personal needs and biases. Rational thinking minus intuition resembles the proverbial rower with only one oar in the water. Rational thought alone only goes around in circles of its own limitations. Breathwalk

stimulates us so we can have both oars in the water and row straight toward mental vitality.

3. FOCUS AND DIRECTED ATTENTION. The ability to quickly bring our minds to peak performance comes up frequently for people in executive roles. But we all can use this capability. Real focus and the ability to rapidly direct our attention depends upon the capacity to let go of whatever has bound up our attention. It also depends on our ability to keep unwanted thoughts and distractions from getting a foothold in our minds. Let them go, and let it flow. Switching the breath can very effectively refocus attention. Patterning the breath in a Breathwalk helps the release of sticky thoughts. It develops our capacity for a neutral mind. A neutral mind lets us refocus.

4. LEARNING AND CREATIVITY. Learning and creativity involve perception—taking in new information, critical assessments and intuitive understandings, action decisions, and careful reassessments of results. A well-done, mindful Breathwalk will free us from old ruts and open us to new information and creativity.

Enjoying a Breathwalk as a routine once a day for five or more times a week can give you a new range of mental vitality and enhanced clarity and focus. The Breathwalk to help enhance each of these qualities is in the guide at the back of this book.

Benefit 4. Feelings of Connectedness

Vitality in body, mind, and spirit requires a strong sense of connectedness. Connectedness is when we feel part of something larger than our normal self. We go beyond our selves and connect with other people, family, and community. We don't just "network" or "check in," we create a real moment of rapport and communication. We feel that the other person is as real to us as our own selves. Connectedness also means going beyond ourselves and connecting with nature. Nature helps us break the isolation that comes from focusing solely on work and a few habitual hangouts. A connection with nature keeps our horizons open and our feet on the ground. It's an antidote for an inflated sense of ego.

Connectedness also means being part of something larger than our mind and its thoughts. We have a connection to spirit, to a vastness that is present and responsive. When we invite that connection in, we are enriched and deepened. Finally, real connectedness begins with a relationship to our true selves. Beyond our impulses, reactions, and personality, there is a self in us that holds our core values and our primary feeling of existence. Being connected to that self helps give us meaning, motivation, and the ability to act with integrity.

You can determine how connected you feel by imagining yourself at the center of a circle. Everything inside that circle feels real and connected to us. If we live within a small radius of connection, our circle includes very few people or things. With a very small radius, we feel connected only to our own impulses and imagination, and we act accordingly: we have few things to compare our feelings and thoughts to. We have a narrow context, and we tend to react from impulse, instinct, and attachments as other animals in nature do. With a bigger radius, our circle reaches out in all directions. We feel connected to a large number of other people and to their minds and feelings; we begin to experience the many dramas, conflicts, and gray areas of feelings that mix opposites like kindness with pettiness, sadness with joy, and love with anger.

Then sometimes our heart center opens wide and we are able to extend the radius of connection even farther than we could imagine. This opening can happen through awareness produced by meditative breathing. We go beyond the normal, everyday experiences of life and begin feeling connected to all other minds, to our own souls, and to the universe. We are still at the center of a circle, but the circle has an infinite radius. Each of our actions and thoughts is connected to the universe. We become intuitive and sense the play of action and reaction in our relationships and in the world. We become vital, secure, flexible, and aware.

The level of connectedness we feel directly impacts the quality of our relationships—all of them. Disconnected, we can feel needy and dependent. We look to others to fill the gap, the loneliness we sense inside of us. We can become controlling since we feel that controlling another person will relieve the isolation we feel inside ourselves. Another reaction to the feeling of disconnection is to form an idea of ourselves that is self-centered, narcissistic, or arrogantly entitled. These unhealthy attitudes develop quite naturally when we are disconnected or live in a radius of connection that is far too small for our mind and soul.

Connectedness, on the other hand, extends our relationships out from us like spokes on a great wheel. That connectedness brings resources, belonging, and the need for many skills like rapport and clear communication. It brings feelings of abundance instead of scarcity and love instead of simply attachment.

Given the nature of connectedness, it should not be surprising that recent research supports its importance and confirms our common sense about its impact. For adolescents, connectedness has emerged as the major protective factor against emotional disturbance, violence, substance abuse, and sexual misconduct. An article in the September 10, 1997, issue of the *Journal of the American Medical Association* concluded in a national survey that there is "consistent evidence that perceived caring and connectedness to others is important in the health of young people today. . . . Parent-family connectedness and perceived school connectedness were protective against every health risk. . . ." Other studies have shown when we come down with a cold, those who have six or more positive social connections recovered four times more quickly than those who had fewer than four social ties. Study after study has found that a strong feeling of connectedness and a diverse and numerous social network protect us against mental and physical illness and create more sustained success and happiness.

Dr. Ed Hallowell, a psychiatrist at Harvard and an advocate of our need to pay attention to our connectedness, makes the importance clear in his 1999 book, *Connect: 12 Vital Ties That Open Your Heart, Lengthen Your Life, and Deepen Your Soul.* After many years of practice he has concluded, "It is time for the message to make its way from the medical and scientific journals into the minds of us all. Connectedness is essential for emotional and physical health at all ages. . . . Many of the young people who sought treatment for depression had achieved high levels of material success but felt depressed because they had not connected in a significant way to anything larger than themselves . . . to one another, to a loved one, to an ideal, or to a purpose or group they believed in. . . . As the years have passed, I have seen the trend only deepen. People are increasingly working at home or working in isolation at their jobs . . . according to the prevailing needs of the new, knowledge-based economy, but all the while feeling more insecure, cynical, worried and finally, isolated." (pp. 9–10)

Connectedness is one of the first things to disintegrate as we get mentally or physically ill. It is one of the highest benefits of being vital and balanced in body, mind, and spirit. That is partly because forming and maintaining a connected relationship is one of the most complex things that we do. We connect with a person by what we say and by an enormous range of nonverbal cues. When we talk to each other, our entire body and our breathing move in orchestrated rhythms. Our relationships are maintained as much by unconscious feelings and cues as by our conscious ones. There is an entire scientific discipline devoted to the study of how we find rapport and bond with one another.

As Dr. Hallowell points out, our new environments in the knowledge economy, our extensive mobility, and the constant pressure to perform well interfere with rapport building and connectedness. That leaves us unprotected and open to a host of maladies. Cybervillages have not replaced the human contact of a physical village or a direct meeting with friends. In fact, a recent study showed a direct correlation between the number of hours people spent on the Internet and depression. This is not a problem with the Internet itself. It has become a problem because people decreased their contacts with others while using the Internet. We need to build in good connectedness as part of effective behavior for living in an information-intensive environment.

There is a solution to the problem. We *can* increase connectedness and its several dimensions. It is one of the four main benefits of doing Breathwalk. The first impact is on ourselves. It begins with us even though the feeling of connectedness we get ultimately helps us to form connections with others, nature, and our spirit. As we bring energy and change to ourselves, we open the way to connect better with others. Initially focusing on ourselves leads us to the capacity to go beyond ourselves.

Breathwalk does this by giving us energy. By breaking old patterns in our body that keep us out of synch and rapport with others, it provides the opportunity for interaction with nature, ourselves, and others as we elevate our mood and sharpen our senses. Breathwalk's gradual pace steadily brings together all of our parts so we are ready to connect. Because we use our meditative mind as we walk in Breathwalk, the exercise connects us to our inner self. It is only as we become thoroughly connected to the inner self that we can connect in authentic ways to others, to nature, and to our spirit. Listen to the following example.

John and Kelly are married and work together in their massage and healing practice. After fifteen years of marriage and eight years of running their business together, communication between them had reached an all-time low. After a Breathwalk workshop they committed to a half-hour walk at noontime and a half-hour walk at the end of each workday. They took the walks together. They tried various Breathwalk patterns and used the Innerwalk techniques extensively. Almost immediately John and Kelly noticed a feeling of connection to each other as they sat in silence at the end of their walks. Gradually they discovered that they had been more drained at the end of each day than either had understood. After the Breathwalks revived their energy levels, it helped them to talk "as if we were on the same planet." They solved the rifts between them and even engaged in ten weeks of brief therapy to act on their insights. Now they do a Breathwalk every day at their clinic and told us, "We come back in the afternoon and immediately connect with our patients. I think half of the healing is the good bedside manner and healing aura that we have after we tune in to each other on our walks."

As we expand our radius of connections and direct ourselves to connect to those feelings, others automatically sense this and try to connect with us even more. We need never manipulate anyone into a relationship. When we are connected to ourselves, we generate a charisma and genuineness that act like a magnet. It is as if the universe asks for our openness to connect and then brings us many opportunities for connection.

There are four main parts to the state of connectedness that secures its many positive effects. Breathwalk effectively strengthens each of them. They are rapport, consistency, integrity, and presence. When these are strong in us, relationships and forming connections become easy.

Four Elements of Connectedness

1. OUT OF RAPPORT SHIFTED TO RAPPORT. To connect with one another, we need to be on the same wavelength. If one person acts as if she just consumed six cups of coffee and the other appears ready for sleep, a fundamental disconnect occurs. All the nonverbal cues will be off. The speed and tone of their language will not match. We all take on rhythms that match our activities. If we return from work high-strung, then we may need to calm down in order to establish rapport with our mate at home. Or we may return from a vacation travel experience and need to adjust ourselves in order to synchronize emotionally and mentally with an energized colleague at work. Much of the art of relationships

comes from putting our entire body and mind into a rhythm and energy level similar to those of our partner. We'll give you some Breathwalk patterns to do just that.

2. INCONSISTENCY SHIFTED TO CONSISTENCY. If your hands feel relaxed and want to reach out but your feet wiggle up and down as if on a race, you're giving out a mixed message. This inner inconsistency sends an immediate alert to other people. We suddenly lose our credibility and the power to let our words and feelings penetrate to the other person. Consistency among our inner parts and across our senses and body is essential to connectedness and the vitality that comes with it.

3. NON-INTEGRITY SHIFTED TO INTEGRITY. Integrity arises from acting on the core feeling of wholeness in our selves. When we speak to others from our whole selves, we communicate honestly and discharge our feelings without ruse or guise. Then we project integrity. Our communication connects with heart and soul. The other person feels that inner connection in our speech and our manner. Nothing can better connect us to another person.

4. DETACHMENT SHIFTED TO EMOTIONAL PRESENCE. The other person whom we want to relate to wants us to be emotionally present—available both to express and empathize with authentic feelings. Emotional presence comes from a combination of inner centeredness, forgiveness of others, and sensitivity. Spiritual presence comes from our radiance, neutral mind, and willingness to see the infinite in the other person. Breathwalk—with its powerful effects upon mood, feelings, and mind—is a versatile tool for creating presence.

At the end of each Breathwalk, take the time to sense your state of connectedness. It is not difficult to expand this, and there is no reason to feel disconnected. You can try the Breathwalks described in the guide at the back of this book for each of these four areas and for the overall feeling of connectedness. It is part of the vitality that springs from life itself.

This detailed tour of the four main beneficial states Breathwalking produces should have given you a good idea of the kinds of experiences you want to create with your Breathwalks. Whether you walk for fun, to stabilize your weight, to be social, or to explore nature, you can get all these benefits and enhance your resources in the area you choose at the same time. Exercise, breathing patterns, and a meditative attitude take you a long way past calorie counting and aerobic benefits. These benefits are certainly a part of the Breathwalk program, but you will also increase the glow of vitality and the radiance of a clear mind. Every benefit, small and large, that we have described in this tour has a direct Breathwalk pattern that can enhance it.

Points to Remember

- We possess vast "underground" sources of energy— in our breath and in our musculature and glands— ready to be tapped and used. Breathwalk connects us with these underutilized energy sources.
- Our minds and our bodies both hold energy in the form of tension and attention. Release tension and direct attention, and we summon up vast new energy sources.
- We experience our personal energy in three common qualities: quick start energy, core energy, and gathered energy. Breathwalk exercises help build up all three to give you vitality.
- Invincible vitality is more than energy; it comes from the alignment of all forms of our energy using body, mind, and spirit.
- Mood states can be switched from negative to positive through the right physical actions combined with breath and attention.
- Not learning to change your mood to support what you want to do bears a high cost economically, physically, and socially.
- The four most common upset mood states and their shifts to healthy opposites are simple anxiety shifted to inner calm; depressed shifted to clear and connected; distracted, busy, and hyperactive shifted to receptive and intimate; and doubtful and lethargic shifted to motivated and ready.
- We can increase our choices about moods if we use

body and mind together with the power of the breath.

- Four qualities of the mind come with real mental vitality: mental clarity, intuition, focus and directed attention, and learning and creativity.
- The mind can become either our most faithful servant or our worst master. Conquer your own mind, and you conquer the world.
- Connectedness is a primary protector against illness and emotional imbalances. Its impact is often underestimated.
- The state of connectedness has four areas we need to manage for real vitality: rapport, consistency, integrity, and emotional presence. Use Breathwalk to bring each of these four areas to the positive side of their polarities, and your relationships will glow with health and good communication.
- Connectedness is when we can be part of something greater than our normal selves. Rapport and integrity with our selves is the beginning of all forms of connectedness.

2

Breathing for Vitality

THE EXTENSIVE AND SOPHISTICATED USE of conscious breathing distinguishes Breathwalk from other approaches to walking and exercise. It is one of the primary reasons we can create so many specific and powerful experiences. We can vary the experience of a walk in dozens of ways with a small alteration in the pattern of breathing. We can refine that even more as we adjust both the awakener exercises in the first step and the way we direct our attention in the last step of the Breathwalk.

The effectiveness of Breathwalk rests on the inseparable link between body and mind through the breath. This link gives us the tools to create healthful changes and powerful experiences. We can work on mind and emotions through the body, and we can affect the body through our breath and awareness.

When we breathe we don't just pump air in and out of our lungs. We send a message coded in the pattern of the breath to the central brain. We trigger changes in the part of our nervous system called the "autonomic nervous system." That's the system that automatically governs such basic things as heart rate and blood pressure and affects some nervous system, glandular, and digestive functions— as well as our breath rate itself. We can think of all the various parts of our bodies and minds as instruments in an orchestra. To get the best harmony and produce the moods and energy we want, we need a conductor. A little area in the lower central brain acts like the conductor. It is called the "hypothalamus." It collects information and signals from the senses, our internal parts, and our emotions. It interacts with all the other areas of the brain. Then it commands the rhythm and quality of our physiology and mind by sending hormones and other signals to the pituitary and other glands in the body. This small area orchestrates the whole cosmic dance and rhythm in our life. It modulates reactions in our immune system, perception, moods, and autonomic functions.

With consciously controlled breathing, we can send coded messages to that inner conductor like scores of music. This will direct our internal state to adjust and change. When we inhale deeply and consciously we actually send a command to the hypothalamus to prepare our whole being for awareness and action. The hypothalamus quietly, silently obeys without question, and millions of electrical and chemical signals race through our bodies like musical notes in a perfect score. We never have to think about the momentous changes going on inside; they are built in.

The conscious breathing in Breathwalk can synchronize all the parts of our body and mind to work together to produce amazing changes. We can release capabilities that have lain dormant. We can become more aware, alert, and healthy. That power resides within us, in our breath. It is our breath's many patterns of variable ratios, frequencies, depth, and other qualities that are the secret code of our nervous system.

What's Wrong with Our Breathing?

Both thinking and feeling stand upon the foundation of breath. Breathe right—and think more clearly. Breathe right—and we create vitality in body, mind, and spirit. Surprisingly, though, many of us breathe wrong. When we do, we gradually lose the harmonious synchronization of our body, mind, and spirit. We slip away from the zone of vitality and from our passion for life and what we do. Our breathing is both automatic and learned. It reflects what we do and how we have felt. So it is very useful to regularly take our breathing off automatic pilot and take charge of it consciously. When we do that we both tune it up and attune ourselves.

Good breathing requires that three movements work together in a proper sequence to maximize the filling and emptying of the lungs. It may sound ridiculously simple, but in fact about one-third of all adults get it wrong. The most common error is that we try to draw air in with the abdomen while pushing it out with the chest, and vice versa. Physiologists call this "paradoxical breathing"—a paradox because we expand our lungs at the same time we reduce our chest cavity space. Our diaphragm and chest muscles then work at cross-purposes. The result? Fatigue and shortness of breath. Exercising while breathing paradoxically becomes labored and can result in dizziness and a tendency to hyperventilate, with uneven breath or gasping from the mouth. Clearly this will not create vitality or good feelings. For approximately one-third of us, then, if we never take time to consciously breathe and breathe with the correct pattern, we will continue living with a fraction of our real vitality. It's like a dog running on three legs and never knowing it could use all four to be faster, smoother, and happier.

Good breathing also means that we synchronize our breathing to our body motions—especially when doing something strenuous such as exercise or playing athletic games. Here, too, our automatic breathing patterns work at cross-purposes for many of us. We lock up our breathing under physical strain and stress, rather than breathing aligned to our physical exertions. When exercising hard, we unconsciously let our abdominal breathing get out of time. We shift to paradoxical breathing. None of these poor breathing habits helps us. All of them send the wrong codes to the brain. From there, those discordant breathing messages create discord in other parts of our body and mind. Fix it and change happens immediately.

How to Breathe Correctly

Just as learning music begins with the basics of notes, learning vitality for body, mind, and spirit begins with the basics of breath. Good breathing comes first, then conscious breathing, and then patterned breathing.

Usually we breathe on automatic pilot. But if we drop the automatic pilot and take conscious control of our breathing, we can notice the effects immediately. Try a small experiment. What happens when we vary the time we spend inhaling relative to exhaling? You can consciously control this ratio. Try breathing in slowly and deeply and then exhaling rapidly. Try five seconds on the inhale and one to two seconds on the exhale. What happens when you do this? Most people feel a surge of energy.

Now try the opposite breath ratio. Breathe in sharply and then exhale slowly and completely. Most people experience a mild calming effect. We seem programmed to do this automatically when we feel the need to calm ourselves and relax. By consciously using this technique, we can shed stress in a hurry.

Breath contains the oxygen we need, but the life we feel when we breathe powerfully and correctly is more than that. We don't feel just oxygen levels. We feel the level of our emotions, thoughts, and spirit. That is why the ancient Latin and French word for breath was *spiritus*. The proper breath can awaken our connection to life and to our spirit. It can take us into a zone of vitality and aliveness that engages our body, our emotions, our thinking, and our spirit equally.

Breathing and its patterns are central to the physiological codes to the body. Proper breathing can trigger the brain to optimize the glands, nerves, and emotions to work together. That's when we enter the zone of vitality. Our research has shown that it is possible to find markers that let us know we have entered that zone. We call it a "signature of wellness." If you move and breathe in the right patterns for an extended time, that signature of wellness shows up in more and more places—our heartbeat variation, our respiratory patterns, and even in the cycles of chemistry in the blood.

The experience of this is that we breathe life and vitality, not just air. Work done by Dr. Herbert Benson and other researchers has shown that conscious attention changes the impact of the breath. Breathing with and without awareness are different things. When we walk with conscious breathing and attention, our moods elevate, our sense of connection and meaning is stronger, and the healing impact of the exercise is multiplied.

Breathing experts have established through research that complete deep breath breathing offers us a number of real benefits over upper-chest breathing. Complete deep breathing can actually

- give us clarity and calmness.
- reduce stress and anxiety.
- help eliminate toxins trapped in the lungs' cilia (little hairs that move mucus and waste) from pollution around us.
- increase patience and resistance to stress reactions.
- improve blood circulation, especially the venous return to the heart.
- optimize the body's acid/alkaline balance, increasing resistance to bacteria and infections.
- facilitate the working of the sacral pump mechanism that moves spinal fluid essential to the nervous system's health and strength.
- help the flow of energy along the body's meridians (energy pathways like those you see in acupuncture charts).

- build the full penetration and strength of the aura (light body).
- modulate and regularize the body's rhythms related to sleep, digestion, sexual urges, and other core functions.

As we cover the basics of breathing, remember that the goal is to help you feel an increase in your vitality. If your basic automatic pattern of breathing has been incorrect, even by an iota, getting it right will give you enormous positive benefits. Breathe right, and your body and mind regulate themselves almost automatically for normal functioning. Basic living doesn't require special efforts; it is when we want more, we want to excel or to intentionally change ourselves, that extra attention is required.

To keep the breath and our system at peak performance it is best to breathe consciously for a little bit every day. Then we never drift far from being and feeling our best. Good breathing begins with the recognition that the act of breathing itself involves three separate, complex series of movements—all of which need to be timed into just the right sequence.

The Three Parts to a Complete Deep Breath
- Lower or abdominal movement
- Middle or chest movement
- Upper or clavicular movement

A full, deep breath uses all three movements completely and in sequence. It begins on the inhale with an outward movement of the abdomen, proceeds upward to an expansion of the chest cavity, and ends with a lifting of the clavicle, or collarbone, and upper chest. The exhale works in just the opposite order.

To understand how breathing works, imagine for a moment that your chest cavity, which holds your lungs, looks like a big, clear bell jar. Sealed over its open bottom is an elastic rubber sheet. You have probably seen a bell jar when it is used to cover and protect fragile objects in displays. It is a cylindrical glass vessel with a rounded top and an open base. It's also used for high school science experiments to show the effects of air pressure vacuums. So imagine that inside the bell jar, your two lungs are hanging like toy balloons. If we lower the air pressure inside the jar by pulling down on the elastic cover, the balloons will fill with outside air. Press the elastic cover upward, into the jar, and the balloons will empty. Your breathing works the same way. The air pressure inside your chest cavity goes up and down, your lungs fill with fresh, outside air, and then they empty. The main pump for that is your diaphragm, which is a large sheet of muscle under the lungs that moves up and down just like the elastic cover we imagined.

We also change the air pressure to expand and contract the lungs by moving our rib cage. That is the second movement. The third movement, clavicular, works as an extension of the chest movement, slightly expanding the top of the chest cavity. The lungs themselves have no muscles. They are passive and need the help of the diaphragm and chest to function. When someone has an accident and punctures through the chest wall, the lungs just hang there until the hole is plugged and they have help to reinflate.

What can be done about the breathing problems that so many of us have? These problems turn out to have easy remedies as long as we breathe consciously in the right patterns for short amounts of time. Then our bodies and brains use their natural intelligence to learn the correct way and keep doing it even when we aren't consciously thinking

about our br

to do a part

quickly lear

ture, withou

what we're

sciousness t

Breathv

check and

start out b

first—such

master the

the basic n

to our awar

Breathwalk.

Breathwalk

deep breath by letting your
and outward. Inhale deepl
as far as you can, slowl
ward your spine. In
complete deep b
Focus upon br
certain to
mouth—

O
of

Complete Deep Breath

The first and most basic breathing tool is the complete deep breath. It has the three parts to it that we have already identified. On the inhale, it starts in the belly, flows smoothly up to the rib cage, and ends in a slight upward movement of the clavicle, or collarbone, and upper chest—all done in a rhythmically flowing manner. On the exhale, everything simply reverses.

Part One: Freeing the Belly

We can actually breathe using only our belly. Try it if you like. First, seat yourself on a firm chair or on the floor. Let your breathing relax at a normal pace depth. Now, bring your conscious attention down to your navel. Take a slow,

belly relax and move forward
. When you've pushed your belly
exhale by pulling your navel to-
order to isolate just this part of the
eath, keep your chest relaxed and still.
athing entirely with your abdomen. Make
breathe through your nostrils—not your
s you do any of these exercises.

er the years we've taught this basic step to thousands
eople and have come to realize that a frequent source
f difficulty has been our Western cultural training to hold
our stomachs tight and never let our bellies stick out. In this
society we are deeply afraid to look fat. We learn to hold in
the belly, to lock it up and prevent its natural movement.
For complete, natural powerful breathing, free the belly.
When it moves right it helps you take a natural full breath,
it builds reserve energy, and for many people it relieves a
common source of pain in the lower back. The vertebrae in
the spine move more freely and will even self-adjust if your
belly is free to move with your breath. Don't worry about
the belly. The extra energy the breath gives you and the
smooth motion in your gait from breathing right will make
you very attractive.

What happens, of course, is that your diaphragm moves
with your belly, and that causes you to breathe. Your body
has within it a diaphragm that looks like a solid sheet of
muscle separating your chest cavity and lungs from your
abdomen and intestines. It normally has a slightly domed
shape to it. As you extend your belly, you also tighten all
those diaphragm muscles; the diaphragm shape flattens out
a bit, and you create an extra space—a vacuum or low-
pressure area—in your chest cavity. Your lungs expand to
equalize the pressure in your chest cavity; you breathe in.

Pull your belly in, and the opposite thing happens. Your diaphragm returns to a dome shape, creating pressure inside the reduced area of your chest cavity. Your lungs collapse inward; you breathe out. When exhaling, make sure you pull your belly in tightly toward your spine. Otherwise the lower area of your lungs will not empty properly. Then you're not running on your full lung power. Keep it up; just breathe slowly and deeply with your abdomen alone. Notice how relaxing this can be.

If you experience difficulty doing this, try lying on your back. Raise your knees comfortably. Place a book on your belly and your hands across your chest. Now you've got two ways to tell you how you're doing. Your hands will assure you that your chest remains still. The book marks the movement of your belly. Push your belly out now; raise that book as high as you can. You'll feel yourself inhaling air. Don't move your chest, though. Now lower the book. Feel yourself exhaling air as the book lowers and the navel pulls back toward the spine. Now you can tell visually just how your conscious, deep abdominal breathing is working. Notice the way that only your abdominal muscles are working; everything else remains still. With a little practice you will master this if it's not already correct.

Part Two: Expanding Your Chest

This time, sit straight and keep your diaphragm still. Don't let your navel area move. Instead use your chest muscles to expand your rib cage. Concentrate upon your rib cage. Now, expand it—make it grow larger, as large as you comfortably can. Soon you can actually feel the intercostal muscles between your ribs pushing and rotating your rib cage outward and upward. Concentrate upon sensing your expanding chest cavity and rotating ribs.

Notice how the depth and volume of your breathing now compares to abdominal breathing. Your breathing diminishes without the abdomen at work. Of course, that's why paradoxical breathing rapidly becomes self-defeating. In paradoxical breathing your chest muscles and diaphragm muscles work against one another, nearly canceling each other out.

Also notice how complicated chest breathing really is; it's a sequence that moves many little parts and connections to your rib cage and spine, instead of just moving a single large sheet of muscle. In reality, most of the potential expansion of our lungs comes from the pressure change powered by the diaphragm. Expanding the chest and adjusting the ribs add a little more space and encourage the full inflation of the lung sac.

Part Three: Moving the Collarbone and Upper Chest

Now let's disengage abdominal and chest breathing for a moment. Sit up straight once more. Pull in the navel slightly and hold it there. This disengages the abdomen. Lift your chest and shoulders slightly without inhaling. Now, inhale slowly by lifting your collarbone and upper chest while moving your shoulders back a bit. Exhale slowly by reversing the order as you keep your midchest lifted. On the exhale, the collarbone drops and the shoulders move forward. You can actually feel a slight motion to breathe while doing this, very slight. You can also figure out pretty quickly that this sort of breathing alone just won't do. It will, however, add that last little bit of filling and emptying to the lungs when you really need maximum lung capacity.

Now that you know each area involved in complete breathing, let's combine them into complete deep breathing. Again, seat yourself on a firm chair or the floor with a straight spine. Begin to inhale with your abdomen. Then, add chest breathing as your belly expands. When your belly gets fully extended outward and your chest feels expanded, add clavicular breath. To exhale, reverse the process. First, relax your clavicle and upper chest. Then, let the midchest relax and smoothly begin to pull in your abdomen. It becomes a smooth, wavelike pulse, in and out—like ascending and descending a primary music scale. Keep it up, in a rhythmic manner. Notice how good it feels and how your flow of thoughts and feelings change.

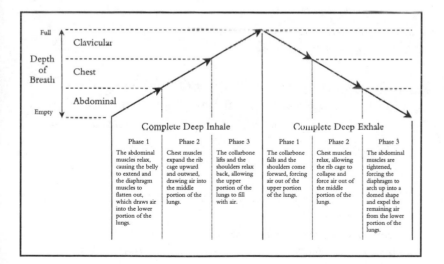

Fixing Some Common Breathing Faults

Here are some of the most common breathing faults and how to fix them:

Jerky Breathing

Each part of the breath comes separately rather than flowing together naturally. Cause: Trying too hard. A simple fix: Put a finger about four inches in front of your torso. As you breathe, move your finger smoothly up and down, from the level of your navel to your chin. Let this be the "conductor's baton" that you concentrate upon as you breathe, raising the "baton" as you inhale and lowering it as you exhale.

Tightening the Shoulders During Clavicular Breathing

This tends to pull the shoulders forward and lessens the space for breathing. Cause: Tension. A simple fix: Flex your shoulders to relax the muscles. Focus your conscious efforts upon your abdomen and chest.

Reverting to Paradoxical Breathing

You start breathing correctly but slip back to the old pattern. Cause: Lack of practice. A simple fix: Practice in short intervals of three to five minutes. Give your full attention to the pattern of the breath until you can simply feel it. Once you can feel the flow of movement and the pleasure of a full breath, your brain will learn it, remember it, and continue it when you are not paying attention.

A Conscious Deep Breathing Exercise

Here's a breath awareness exercise to help you gain peak performance. Do it anywhere, anytime you feel you need a boost—for instance, during a busy, stress-filled day. Even if you only have three to five minutes of personal time, you can slip into your zone of vitality and clarity so you can work at your best for the remainder of the day. You might do this during a short break from work, sitting at your desk or anywhere else you can sit undisturbed for three minutes up to one hour.

Sit with your spine erect, resting your hands on your lap, palms up and fingers slightly curled, right hand into the left with your thumbs touching. Close your eyes. Feel your body come to perfect balance. Sit without effort; equalize the weight on your thighs and hips. That way you center your navel point and properly adjust your breathing motion.

Now focus all of your conscious attention on your own breathing. Breathe through your nose. Notice your breath's flow, the sensations you feel as it courses in and out of your nostrils. Sense the motion and energy your breath has, as if it is very much alive and can travel all over your body. How does it seem to move in the various parts of your body? Is it quick and fiery all over your body or slow and poky in some areas? Is it light and ticklish or smooth and dark?

Concentrate totally upon the breath flowing through your body. Pay careful attention. How does the flow of breath change as a result of the attention you pay to it?

After one or two minutes bring your attention to the one square inch on your forehead just above the root of your nose—the brow point. Survey your entire body from the brow point. Then focus on one area—the navel point. The experience is like standing at the top of a hill and from that vantage point surveying all the land around you before focusing in on one beautiful orchard in the distance. Do a long, slow, complete deep breath. Feel your breath's motion throughout your body connected to the pulse from your navel. Sense the waves of motion that emanate from your navel with this complete deep breath.

Visualize your body as luminous. See each cell acquire a little glow. Notice your entire body shining with a light many feet around it. Be cozy, bright, and conscious. Continue to breathe consciously, but gradually let your breath breathe you. Let the breathing become effortless, and stay fully aware. Sense your breath as a wave in the much greater ocean of breath that you are a part of. Feel the pulse of Life itself. Breath is a gift. From your first gasp as a baby to this moment, breath runs through you as the thread of life. Now build up your relationship to all the sensations of your breath, including the feeling of life and your gratitude for life. Arouse every part of your brain by establishing a living relationship to your breath. The natural flow of complete deep breath will pass through every cell of your being. You can begin to vividly sense your center, your awareness, your baseline of energy, and your mood.

Continue this way for between three and sixty-two minutes. You will improve your breathing, calm yourself, and develop sensitivity to your own state and condition. Well before we become conscious of many illnesses or emotional upsets, our brain registers sensitive imbalances in the subtle motions and feelings of breath flowing throughout the body. By attending to complete breathing in this manner, you become open to the messages of the conscious and unconscious realms of mind and emotions. This conscious deep breathing will begin to attune you to your vitality and to the flows in your life.

Points to Remember

- We breathe for life and vitality as much as for air.
- Over 30 percent of us breathe incorrectly and rob ourselves of vitality. It is easy to correct with a little practice of conscious breathing in the proper pattern.
- A complete deep breath is a single flowing motion with three parts to it: abdominal, chest, and clavicular.
- Good breathing sends a code to the brain that helps adjust a wide range of ailments and open a treasury of benefits.
- We should breathe consciously on a daily basis to keep our breath pattern strong since it is subject to our emotions and habits.
- Breathwalk uses both basic and refined breathing patterns to give us maximum vitality in our lives.

3 The Breath's Code—Sending Signals to Your Body and Mind

So far, you have learned the most basic practice of complete deep breathing. This is not all; breathing has even more dimensions to it. The next five practices involve breath suspension, changed frequencies, ratios, segments, and rapidity of breathing. These additional dimensions to breathing are as basic as an alphabet. They will allow you to send sophisticated and specific patterns of instructions, like a code, to the hypothalamus triggering your body and mind to shift into states of your choice—energy, mental clarity, positive moods, and more.

In the last chapter we introduced you to

consciously controlled breathing—long, deep, and complete breaths. You could breathe that way through a normal day and do just fine. So why learn to breathe other ways? Well, imagine just strolling. You can get most places and enjoy the outdoors with that stroll. But what if you want to cover ground quickly? Then you run. Or you want to reach a high tree branch. Then you jump. Or you may need to cross over a roiling stream. Then you leap. For special purposes we need to learn special patterns of breathing as well as walking that fit the challenge of the moment.

As you learn the various patterns of breathing and their effects on your mind and body, you will improve your range of choices of how to take control of your life energy. When you can match your energy to the task you want to accomplish or the challenge you face, you can feel more confident, powerful, and relaxed. We need a strong focused energy with maximum alertness when we have a competitive challenge basketball. We need a quieter, more receptive state when we meet to negotiate a business deal or a new mortgage. When we want to reach a place of maximum rapport and connection with someone, we want playful energy, both expressive and clear. Having a way to quickly and confidently get to the state you need is a potent ally for success and enjoyment. In this chapter you will be introduced to some new patterns of breathing that are a little uncommon. These different methods of breathing are easy to learn but may be unlike any feeling you have experienced before. With these breathing practices you will have the tools needed to command your own state.

Suspending the Breath

During Breathwalks we often suspend the breath briefly after an exercise or after taking a deep breath in order to integrate and distribute the effects through the entire body. Many people when they are first introduced to breath suspension see it as simply holding their breath. We prefer the term "suspending the breath"; you gently, momentarily cease the mechanism of breathing and become still in body and mind. What's the big difference between this and "holding" your breath? If we say "hold it," many people just tighten their muscles to force the breath to stop. They lock muscles, fight against the breath, and become tense. This defensive posture is not what we mean by breath suspension, which is a gentle, graceful art. Suspending stops your breathing, not by creating an opposition in your muscle groups, but by gently relaxing the whole breathing musculature—the muscles of the diaphragm, ribs, and abdomen responsible for all breathing motion in the first place.

When you hold your breath the wrong way with your chin pulled in, your neck and throat muscles crunched tightly together, and your tongue stiffened, you create great pressure in the eyes, the back of the skull, the heart, and the neck. Done for more than a few seconds, this homespun technique can lead to dizziness, headaches, and vascular difficulties in your eyes. And if you continue to hold your breath improperly, you will train your subconscious to repeat the mistake when you are not aware of it—in moments of fear, anger, and anxiety. Your body's learned patterns can lead you to problems instead of benefits. On the other hand, by training your subconscious correctly, you can continue to help your body suspend breath and breathe correctly even when you are not paying attention.

Sitting with your spine upright, inhale deeply. Bring your conscious attention to your clavicle and ribs. Now lift your upper ribs slightly and fix them in place. Done right, it feels as if a hook has grabbed the center of your breastbone, lifting it up and out a bit. Now relax your shoulders; relax your belly. Notice how easy it becomes to hold your diaphragm steady once you relax your belly outward. Finally, pull your chin in. Become still and calm. No motion, no breathing. The breathing musculature has come to a halt. You have now suspended your breath on an inhalation. Pause for a bit, and then gently resume normal breathing

How long should you suspend your breath in this manner? Don't worry, your brain will trigger you to breathe when the carbon dioxide level of your blood rises too high. When your carbon dioxide buildup urges you to breathe, exhale gently. If you begin to feel a slight dizziness, stop suspending your breath! Dizziness will not help tune up your nervous system.

To suspend your breath exhaled, start with a complete exhale. Let the upper ribs relax and compress. Then pull your navel point back toward your spine. Lift up your chest, lock in the chin comfortably, and keep the navel pulled in firmly but without strain. Become calm and still like a boat that has just cut its engine and now glides peacefully over the calm surface of a lake. If you find your muscles starting an inhalation reflex, simply consciously exhale a little more—shoot out a puff of breath in a quick stroke through your nose and suspend your chest again. In this way you can extend your breath suspension significantly without any strain or struggle.

When you suspend your breath in this manner, you

will cause a shift in your metabolic activity, in your nervous system balance, and in your mood. Practicing breath suspension as a consciously controlled exercise will create a calm internal spot in your awareness. You will begin to notice healthful changes in your body and mind. Your body will begin to work at higher levels of efficiency. Breath suspension will impact your emotional brain, and you will find that it has a calming effect upon your moods. Breath suspension will also train you to use good judgment under pressure—something we all need in our lives.

A well-done breath suspension has three major impacts: centering, distributing, and integrating. Emotions and thoughts become centered; jumpiness and distraction stops. The energy that you developed in your exercise, Breathwalk, or meditation seems to flow freely to every area of your body. It refreshes you like a mist going to every thirsty plant during a gentle rainfall. Last, the suspension integrates the actions of your organs and muscles. During the stillness and quietude of the suspension, the signals between them are sharper and received more clearly, just the way an orchestra becomes still when the conductor appears so the musicians can all hear each other and work together.

Breath Frequency

When you consciously lower the rate at which you breathe in and out, you gain many healthful body and mind benefits. Breath frequency is nothing more than the number of times per minute that we do a complete breathing cycle of inhale and then exhale. Normally men breathe at a rate of sixteen to eighteen cycles per minute, women eighteen to twenty, and children twenty to twenty-six. Infants normally breathe much faster—thirty to thirty-five cycles per minute. Few of us ever bother to think about what happens when we consciously choose to breathe more slowly. The impact may surprise you.

Sit once more with your spine erect and do some complete deep breathing. You are probably breathing at twelve cycles per minute or more. Now consciously lower your breathing frequency to eight cycles per minute. Breathe fully and deeply enough to reach a comfort level at this slower breath frequency. Continue for fifteen minutes. Keep your conscious attention focused on your flow of breath and flow of thoughts. At this frequency of breathing, you alert your body and brain to adjust to the change and to open your lungs as you relax the body. You begin to feel less stressed and more aware. The movement from normal breathing to breathing at a rate of eight cycles per minute has alerted the brain and started a gradual healing process. After fifteen minutes return to normal breathing. You may note that your skin, the entire surface and boundary of your body, actually feels different. Your eyes see more clearly. Your mind has shifted to a different mode. The thoughts that stay with you change, and you find you can let go of feelings and thoughts that seemed persistent before. You feel intensely aware. Additional parts of your brain and your endocrine system have become engaged in the healing effects you now experience.

Try this practice again, this time reducing the frequency to four cycles per minute. Check the results when you've completed the fifteen-minute experiment. If you like these results, try the slowest breath rhythm: one cycle per minute. The best way to do this is to inhale slowly and consciously for twenty seconds. Then suspend your breath for twenty seconds. Finally release the breath gradually and evenly for twenty seconds. Immediately restart the cycle. If you could do this breath every day for thirty-one minutes at a time, that would change your life. It boosts the immune system, puts you in command of your impulses, and creates a pressure to optimize the two sides of your brain to work together harmoniously.

A Table of Breathing Frequencies and Their Impacts

Breath Frequency	Health Impacts
8 cycles per minute	Relief from stress and increased mental awareness.
4 cycles per minute	Positive shifts in mental function, intense feelings of awareness, increased visual clarity, heightened bodily sensitivity.
1 cycle per minute	Optimized cooperation between brain hemispheres, dramatic calming of anxiety, fear, and worry. Intuition expands. Openness to feeling your own presence and the presence of spirit.

Breath Ratios

A breath ratio is simply the amount of time you spend inhaling compared to the amount of time you spend exhaling. When we breathe automatically we tend to breathe in equal timing—in and out, in and out. Now, think consciously about a difference between your inhalation time and exhalation time. You actually can breathe in unequal as well as equal ratios. You might, for instance, inhale very slowly and exhale sharply. You move the same volume of air, only the rate at which you move it changes. A simple diagram helps you actually see the difference.

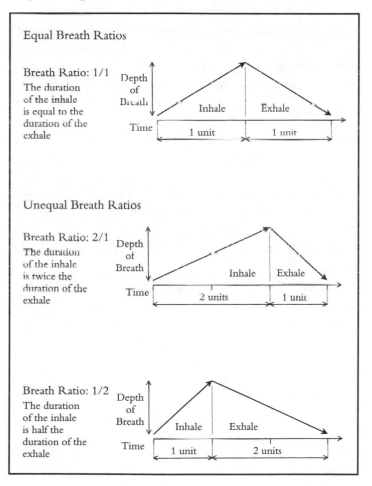

Equal Breath Ratios

Breath Ratio: 1/1
The duration of the inhale is equal to the duration of the exhale

Depth of Breath

Inhale | Exhale

Time | 1 unit | 1 unit

Unequal Breath Ratios

Breath Ratio: 2/1
The duration of the inhale is twice the duration of the exhale

Depth of Breath

Inhale | Exhale

Time | 2 units | 1 unit

Breath Ratio: 1/2
The duration of the inhale is half the duration of the exhale

Depth of Breath

Inhale | Exhale

Time | 1 unit | 2 units

You may remember that you have already encountered such a difference in the simple practice given on page 55. There you performed one unequal breathing cycle and found out its effects. We all do this without even thinking about it. Inhale more slowly before facing a challenge; exhale more slowly to relax. You could, of course, keep on breathing in an unequal ratio for a much longer time.

When you do this, you find that unequal breath ratios work to vary the amount of energy available for the body to use. The key seems to lie in the way the autonomic nervous system responds to such breathing rhythms. Just as the rhythms of your legs when walking work as a vibrating pendulum, so too does your breathing. Both breathing and walking work like a musical metronome that your body and mind follows. When you emphasize inhaling over exhaling, the sympathetic part of the autonomic nervous system boosts your heart rate and blood pressure. When you emphasize exhaling over inhaling, the parasympathetic part slows your heartbeat and relaxes the circulation, nerves, and digestive system. Together the sympathetic and parasympathetic systems work rather like the accelerator and brakes in your car.

Varying your breath ratio has some important practical uses. Changing the ratio can make you warm or cold; it can nourish body tissue; it can alter your sleep pattern and your flow of thoughts. It can help or hinder your adjustment to time zone shifts and sudden disruptions in your schedule. It can change basic processes such as the clotting of your blood, the healing of bruises, and the strength of your immune system response to infections and stress.

Segmented Breathing

Segmented breathing means dividing each inhalation and exhalation that we take into several equal parts, with a slight breath suspension separating each part. As such, segmented breathing is a dynamic use of breath suspension applied to complete deep breathing. In the dynamic process of full breathing itself, we introduce slight pauses in a regular, rhythmic fashion. Unlike our other breathing tools, segmented breathing has no natural counterpart. It represents a distinct, totally conscious style. Visually, segmented breathing looks like the following diagram.

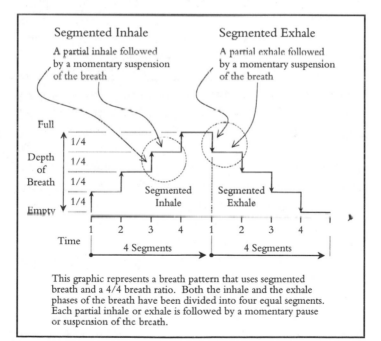

This graphic represents a breath pattern that uses segmented breath and a 4/4 breath ratio. Both the inhale and the exhale phases of the breath have been divided into four equal segments. Each partial inhale or exhale is followed by a momentary pause or suspension of the breath.

Here's how to begin segmented breathing. Instead of inhaling in one smooth stroke, try inhaling in four equal segments, each broken by a very momentary pause or breath suspension. Do the same thing exhaling. You'll find that this breathing pattern combines beautifully with walking. You can time your breath segments to your walking stride.

Begin developing your skill with this tool by concentrating upon making all the segments of your breathing—both inhaling and exhaling—the same. No unequal breath ratios. No holding your breath at the end of an inhalation or exhalation—just smooth, equal parts. Start by consciously separating your breath into four equal segments, in and out—in 4/4 time, just like a beat in music. Work at performing this exercise so the entire cycle is like a complete, deep breath—but accomplished in parts. You may also wish to try 8/8 time once you've mastered 4/4 time. Remember always to breathe through the nose.

As you segment your breathing, make the pressure of your breath strike a comfortable place in your air passages, usually the mid- to top nose area. When you sniff your breath in, or inhale, you can feel the pressure of the air on the tip of your nose. Sniff too hard, and chances are you will begin to squeeze your nostrils together, blocking off the flow of air. Work at relaxing your nose when segmenting your breath, and you'll find that you can easily direct the flow of your breath on the inhale so as to strike farther up into your nose. It's just a matter of regulating how vigorously you breathe. If you pull your breath all the way into your throat or lungs, everything will be too open. Done right, your breath strikes a relaxed but controlled area in your nasal passage that stimulates a special set of nerves. Now, on the exhale, relax your throat area. Regulate exhaling by using navel movement. Pull your navel inward, coordinated with relaxing your chest. When you focus air correctly, segmented breathing feels very natural.

Segmented breathing works by alerting the central brain differently from the way a smooth breath does. Even though you may breathe just as deeply in total volume as in a complete deep breath, and even though the timing of a complete cycle of the breath is the same, the impact differs radically. The accelerated movements of muscle and nerves that let you segment the breath generate a different code and message to the body and mind system. You alert your glands to calibrate themselves and to act optimally. The difference impacts the tone of the endocrine and immune systems of the body. It also makes the nervous system strong under stress. The sum of the parts has become different from, and more than, the whole breath by itself.

This exercise will develop your capacity for segmented breathing while also working to heal your body. Try it now. Make sure that you will be undisturbed for the next five to fifteen minutes. Sit straight in a firm chair or on the floor and close your eyes, focusing upon the brow point.

Begin to inhale, while segmenting your breath into eight equal steps. Now exhale in eight equal steps also. Keep focused upon your breathing. It is like going up and down a ladder with eight rungs. You may wish to repeat mentally the primal sounds as you inhale. Say to yourself SA TA NA MA twice as you inhale and twice as you exhale, one primal sound for each segment to your breath. We will examine the use of sounds later. For now just try them like a do-re-mi scale for the mind. Continue for five to fifteen minutes. At the end, inhale deeply and suspend your breath briefly. Then sit and feel the effects of your breath in every cell of your body. Visually scan each cell and feel that it is well and healed.

Rapid Breathing

The next two techniques use a rapid breath instead of a slow or segmented breath. They are known as the breath of fire and the cannon breath in the tradition of kundalini yoga. They are two techniques with unparalleled ability to restore and rejuvenate the whole body and mind.

Breath of Fire

A dramatic name for a dramatic breathing pattern, this exercise will completely readjust your nervous system and give you nerves of steel. If you learn breath of fire, you can eliminate the most tenacious stress from your being. The breath pattern is simple—rapid breathing through the nose. The rate should be between 120 and 180 strokes per minute. A stroke is one inhalation and exhalation. This is really fast! Your breathing should be continuous and very smooth. Your nostrils should remain relaxed and not squeezed closed by your breathing. To exhale doing breath of fire, expel air by pressing your navel point and solar plexus back toward your spine as you contract your diaphragm. This will feel automatic if you contract your diaphragm rapidly enough. To inhale, relax your abdomen so that your diaphragm extends downward and your breath seems to come in naturally with little effort.

Your chest should stay relaxed and slightly lifted

throughout the breathing cycle. Keep the ratio completely equal. If you inhale too much relative to your exhale, you will become dizzy and feel as if you just drank a gallon of coffee. If you exhale too much, you will slow down and get too serious. When you breathe this rapidly, small changes in the ratio of the inhale and exhale can easily produce big changes in the actual air volume you receive. That is uncomfortable and not sustainable. When you get the ratio equalized, your breath gains a momentum and becomes easy. You find yourself becoming alert, energized, and relaxed—all at once.

Keep the cadence steady. An erratic rhythm will be irritating and risks moving you toward an oxygen imbalance.

Keep your upper chest slightly lifted. Some people, especially paradoxical breathers, work too hard at this. If you're uncertain whether your upper chest remains still during this exercise, place one of your hands on your upper chest and the other hand between your solar plexus and your navel point. The upper hand should remain still while you do the breath of fire. The power comes from below. Your lower palm feels the upper abdomen near your solar plexus pulsating with your breath. If you now move your lower hand beneath your navel point, you will find that almost no movement occurs. The breath of fire, then, is not a lower belly pump. That would be a bellows breath.

Relax your shoulders and lower back. Think of this whole exercise as play instead of work. If you pump your belly or tighten your shoulders, you will eventually feel a constriction in your lower back that tires you. Lift your chest a bit, relax your shoulders, and put on the glimmer of a smile as you enjoy the virile activity that you are engaged in.

People frequently ask if this makes you hyperventilate.

No. We could say it gives you superventilation—great lungs and a powerful breath. If you pump your belly strongly, that would move too much air and create a problem. Or if you get the inhale-exhale ratio out of balance, that would cause a problem. Breath of fire done well can be practiced for as long as thirty-one minutes, still feeling great and with no signs of hyperventilation. Blood tests after such a long exercise interval reveal a stable CO_2 level with the oxygen content slightly raised. Nonetheless, always begin with moderate time periods for each practice when developing any new physical skill, especially breathing.

The Benefits of Breath of Fire
- Stress release
- Expanded lung capacity and vital breath
- Expelled toxins from the lung tissues
- Cleared mucous membranes
- Alertness, energy, and strength
- "Signature of wellness" in your body rhythms, like heartbeat
- Balanced autonomic nervous system
- Loss of addictive impulses

Cannon Breath

If you do a slower breath of fire through your mouth, that is called "cannon breath." Its pace should be 120–130 strokes per minute—about 2 strokes per second. Cannon breath can cleanse and strengthen the parasympathetic nerves very rapidly. It can also do a great job of adjusting all digestive functions. It produces widespread arousal in the brain. Not alarm, just arousal—a readiness to learn and respond.

The key to doing cannon breath correctly is to shape your mouth like a round cannon. Don't purse your lips as though you are giving a kiss, and don't open your mouth into a wide cavern. When your mouth forms a small cannon, the pressure of the breath is in the back of your cheeks and along the top of your tongue. Feel the pressure while you do this exercise to help you get your mouth opening right. Your throat will contain some, but not all, of the pressure. Don't hold your throat tightly. Your neck should be straight, with the chin pulled in just slightly. You can do cannon breath for one to three minutes.

Points to Remember

- Breath suspension. Gently cease, momentarily, the mechanism of breathing and become still in body and mind. It yields very healthful benefits when done by itself. It will cause a switch to get thrown in your metabolic activity and in your nervous system balance, calming your mood.
- Breath frequency. Breath frequency is nothing more than the number of times per minute that we do a complete breathing cycle—inhale and then exhale. Lower the rate at which you breathe in and out, and you'll gain many healthful body and mind benefits.
- Breath ratio. A breath ratio is the amount of time you spend inhaling compared with the amount of time you spend exhaling. Changing the ratio can make you warm or cold; it can nourish body tissue; it can alter your sleep pattern and your flow of thoughts and yield many other benefits.

- Segmented breathing. Segmented breathing means dividing each inhalation and exhalation that we take into several equal parts, with a slight breath suspension separating each part. It combines beautifully with walking for a vitality tune-up. You can time your breath segments to your walking stride. Segmented breathing works its healthful effects by alerting the central brain differently from the way a smooth inhalation-exhalation does.

- Rapid breathing. Breath of fire is a rapid breath at 120–180 cycles per minute. It is excellent to rid the body and mind of stress. It acts as a kind of catalyst for change in each posture it is used with.

4

The Experience of Breathwalk

WORDS CAN'T REPLACE DIRECT EXPERIENCE. To really know and understand the benefits of Breathwalk, you need to give it a try. In the next several chapters we will cover all the basics needed to do it well and enjoy it. But first we need to spend a little time getting your breathing correct, aligning your posture, and learning the use of various breath patterns.

There are five steps to the Breathwalk.

- Step One: Awaken your body and mind with special awakener exercise sets.
- Step Two: Align your walking posture and your awareness.

- Step Three: Vitalize with intervals of synchronized breathing and walking.
- Step Four: Balance as you pace yourself down.
- Step Five: Integrate as you enrich and anchor your experience with an Innerwalk.

If you need one last thought to motivate you to jump in with us for a short Breathwalk, consider this: When we walk properly, walking is an excellent basis for increasing our total fitness. Walking can become the springboard for generally improved physical, mental, and spiritual fitness—real vitality. We now know that walking makes an almost perfect exercise. You can gain aerobic benefits, and it actually works more muscles than moderate running.

Over the years, many studies have shown that walking constitutes the perfect "cross-training" exercise. Its aerobic benefits transfer to running, weight lifting, and many other physical activities. It is the most primal exercise we know. Over thousands of years walking has evolved in a way that links it to many systems in the body such as digestion, the heart and circulation, and even the perceptual organs like the eyes. Walking gives those systems a healthful performance tune-up. The heart is strengthened, circulation improved, peristaltic motions of digestion are adjusted, and perception increases acuity and clarity. That is why many top runners and athletes who used to look down upon the slow pace and low-effort levels of walking now include it as a primary staple in their training programs. Far from being boring, walking can help boost your mood. It has a low injury rate, so you can do it for your entire life.

Going on a Breathwalk

We invite you to come along on an early morning Breathwalk with Gurucharan in the foothills of the Sangre de Cristo Mountains of New Mexico.

As I'm working on this Breathwalk guide, I'm also teaching Breathwalk and yoga at a large gathering here in New Mexico. Over the night, the temperature has dropped down from the previous day's scorching high nineties. It's near dawn and a cool morning breeze has just awakened me from a deep rest. Looking around, my eyes see a panorama of subtle dawn colors as the red earth blends playfully with the sky's pinkish blue tones. The desert's like that. I face a demanding twelve hours of teaching later today, so I welcome the boost I know a good Breathwalk will give me. I put on walking shoes and I am ready to begin.

In my mind, I go through the various Breathwalk options and choose one called the Eagle Breathwalk. I'm still adjusting to the altitude shift in coming here from sea level in Boston, and I want something simple that will give me mental clarity and sharpness for my morning seminar. But before setting out to walk, I do an awakener. That's the first step in a complete Breathwalk, to awaken the body and mind. I've picked an awakener with four quick exercises to energize me and boost the immune system and maybe counter some travel stress as well.

I stand with my palms crossed at my chest and begin breath of fire. I breathe in and out through my nostrils, fast. Equal in and out, about two strokes a second. Getting into the rhythm, I keep the pace steady and focus on the sensations of the breath and its energy. I breathe in precise staccato in-and-out breaths. I felt a little clogged up, but after a minute my breathing passages open up. I smell the sweet scent of sage all around; I hadn't noticed it until now. As I continue breath of fire, my sense of smell blossoms and comes fully alive. Three minutes have gone by. I inhale deeply and hold my breath for fifteen seconds while I tighten every muscle in my body. Now! I exhale all at once through the mouth like a cannon shot. I repeat the last inhale and exhale and relax. A tingling wave runs across my skin. It feels good.

Next, I swing my arms in big circles and feel my chest opening further as my arms pump rhythmically. After a minute I feel warmth in my upper chest and a flush on my cheeks. As I inhale at the end, I'm alert. I feel blood pulsing in my fingertips and my heart slowly increasing its beat. Arms outstretched, now I start to rotate my hands. Work at it and concentrate. It's a real effort! In a few seconds my breath synchronizes with my wrist movements. I feel this one in my shoulders. As I inhale and hold my breath, I feel a rush of energy originating in my navel and passing through the chest to the crown of my head. I feel stable and light and very aware. I let the breath go and relax my arms.

In the next exercise I stretch up mightily, raising my arms high above my head. It feels very good to stretch. Then I relax and let my arms down. And repeat. Breathe in as the arms raise up; exhale as they fall. Each cycle of breath and arms leaves me more grounded and sets me more strongly on my feet. My ribs feel open and relaxed. I'm very present in the moment. I'm eager to walk now, but I want to finish this set of exercises to boost my immune system. So I close my right nostril and breathe through the left side only. Each side gives a different message to the hemispheres of my brain. I start to relax as I breathe. It feels soothing. It feels a little like a slow, pleasant spin on a carousel. The breath relaxes me like a gentle wave all over my body, and my thoughts seem to slow down a bit as well. As I look around, it's like seeing the same old road anew, fresh. Sage, dusty earth, and now the flowers across the way are incredibly vivid.

I start to walk now. My legs shake out a bit; I'm not smooth yet. I scan my body mentally. That's the second step in a Breathwalk—aligning every part of my body with a body scan. My right toe's tagging inward a bit. I adjust my feet a little. Hips loosen up; I sense their natural motion returning. I feel a modest pain in my lower left back. I don't react and tense as I usually do with a pain. Instead I relax and go on to scan my chest and shoulders. As my shoulders loosen, the back pain seems to lessen, and that area joins with the rhythm of the rest of my body. I feel myself dropping into a stride now. My neck loosens and perches my head just right. When I scan my body with my mind's eye, everything responds and aligns.

Now I start to breathe consciously in a specific pattern for the effect I want. This is the heart and soul of Breathwalk—it is step three—vitalize—in the Breathwalk. I begin inhaling in four distinct segments in time with my walking pace. The same when exhaling—four segmented chuffs out timed to four paces of my legs. I am breathing through my nose and synchronizing segmented breathing to each footstep. Now I'm in an easy rhythm; the four-segmented deep breaths in and out are almost automatic. Now, mentally, I begin to repeat to myself four primal sounds, SA, TA, NA, MA. SA, TA, NA, MA. I want to hush the inner noise of my mind and break my patterns of inner talk. I shift my attention to the breath and the inner sounds. At first I concentrate upon my breath, to adjust my ribs and chest. Now I start to breathe more deeply, keeping the segments equal and smooth. The inner sounds take up the rest of my attention. Soon I settle into a constant rhythm, and the sound moves to the front of my attention. SA, TA, NA, MA.

I shift to the feel of my own breathing. Inhaling. Four equal segments. Belly thrusts out, my chest fills; the breath seems to pull me upward as my shoulders rise slightly and drop back to increase the depth of my own breathing. Exhaling. Four equal segments. I focus upon pulling in the navel point a bit. Then the breath pulses—steps in and out as I step forward with my feet. Always four segments. SA, TA, NA, MA. Everything falls into perfect synchrony like the harmony in a concert orchestra.

I start to play my fingertips, to do finger magic. All in rhythm. Touching in sequence each finger on each hand to the thumb. It's a timeless rhythm. Fingers moving rhythmically. SA, TA, NA, MA. I can notice everything around me. Trees, hills, barking dogs, birds taking flight. Everything is graphically distinct and three-dimensional. I am flowing, not just walking. I'm full of energy.

After five minutes I relax my breath and stop doing the segmented conscious breathing. Now I'm walking and breathing normally, my body relaxed and loose. This is part of step three—using vitality intervals. I alternate between patterned breathing and walking with a relaxed breath. Checking my body and my feelings, I especially notice my eyesight. I now see three dimensions more fully than before; the world seems somehow richer in colors and in its sense of space. I'm walking past some great cottonwood trees, and I can see the slowly spiraling cotton balls; they move in space to the wind's currents in astounding clarity. Trees and mountains now appear in crisp depth. Each thing has taken on a more vivid reality. I feel very grateful for this moment.

I keep the primal sound scale going. SA, TA, NA, MA. After three minutes I feel ready for a long haul. I start the 4/4 breath again. A slight hill makes me walk slower, more deliberately. I adjust my breath and breathe deeper with SA, TA, NA, MA. The impact of my steady breath cadence spreads over my face and skin. Warmth. Sensitivity.

Aliveness. I feel the flow of air past my cheeks. I feel myself at the center of all this vital activity. My legs warm and feel as though they can go for days without rest. My mental focus shifts back and forth from primal sounds to sensing the world around me, like a giant pendulum in motion. My whole body warms. Not sweaty, just flushed full.

After ten minutes my lungs seem expansive and open. I feel as though I don't even need to breathe any longer. I have enough vital energy within me. But I keep up the cadence SA, TA, NA, MA. I'm in the present, connected to everything. Now I slow down, relax my breath, and pay attention to everything around me. This is the fourth step—balance. I pace down and bring my attention from inside to outside. After two minutes I do the last step, integrate. I want to keep all this awareness and energy with me through the day. I want to anchor it. I do a simple Innerwalk. As I slow down, I mentally review the path and all the steps I took on this walk. I walk it again in my mind and pay attention to each of my senses one at a time. I let this walk and all its changes imprint itself on my mind. Now I gather all my senses back to this moment. I lean against a convenient tree and breathe very slowly. I mentally guide my breath down along each of my limbs and back. I see myself radiant and balanced.

I end at my house and do three final stretching sequences in a smooth, quick motion. I am ready for this day.

We hope this gives you a good feeling for what the experience of a Breathwalk is like. We know each person has his or her own experience. We know that the different Breathwalk patterns feel very different in their effects. So we invite you to explore.

This is just the beginning. As we examine each of the five parts of Breathwalk in detail in chapters 5 through 9, it will become more natural, more effective, more fun. As we explore the variety of Breathwalk patterns and programs, you can find those that support you and your needs. Gradually you can learn to use Breathwalk on long walks and on brief jaunts. It becomes automatic with less focus on Breathwalk and more on the lift it gives to you and your spirit.

5

AWAKEN—Breathwalk Step #1

MOST OF US FEEL THE NEED TO THOR-
oughly awaken our body and mind when we
first arise in the morning. We need to clear
out mental fog, leftover dreams, and any tension and sluggishness in our body. Circulate
the blood, flush our fluids, and focus our
mind. We all perform our own rituals to
awaken. We stretch, take a shower, and brew a
pot of tea or coffee. We also need to awaken
our body and mind every time we do a thorough exercise routine, whether it is ten minutes long or an hour. Our normal activities
can lull us into a kind of waking sleep, a nar-

row focus where we lose touch with our body and with most of our internal resources.

In Breathwalk we start with awakeners, which shake off any dullness or lethargy and selectively stimulate the functions of our body and mind we want to work on. Awakeners consist of specifically designed sequential movements matched to breathing that balance the whole body. Their impact comes from the order and composition of their motions. They take the place of warm-ups in traditional exercise. Some awakeners globally enhance the effects of exercise in every part of your body. Others target a boost to a specific system of your body, such as your immune system, circulation, or lungs. You can choose the awakener that best suits your needs at the moment. Awakeners also stimulate those specific areas of your body that may need special attention or healing, like back muscles, the spine, or the circulatory system. Awakeners prepare you to do the main part of Breathwalk, which is consciously directed breathing synchronized to walking.

Each awakener works slightly different muscles and areas of your body and brain. That means that varying your awakener can build up every part of your body and mind. Some awakeners work better for stimulation and others for relaxation, some for circulation and others for strength, some for focus and action and others for centering. With a little experimentation and the comments we include with each awakener set, you'll quickly discover which awakeners work best for you.

Nearly every awakener involves the same two key actions—breath priming and sequenced movements. Each awakener starts with one to three minutes of consciously controlled breathing. We call this action "breath priming."

Breathwalk

Each awakener takes you through three to five short exercises done in a specific sequence to build up a targeted impact. You can choose the effect you want upon mood, circulation, muscular tension and flexibility, and the neuroendocrine system within your body.

Priming the Breath

Maybe you remember those old hand water pumps that needed priming with a little water before they would work. Or perhaps if you ever had to siphon something, you know you have to force some fluid through the siphoning tube to get the flow started. Our bodies also need some priming to exercise most effectively. Breath priming means that you take a few conscious breaths to set up the flow of breathing. It flows from the universe to our lungs and from our lungs to every cell. We can increase that flow, redirect it, and refine it. We prime our breath so it can function at a higher level. In the process, we expel old air, clear the linings of the lungs, and stimulate circulation.

Here's how to do breath priming. You'll simply be breathing consciously without any distraction for one to three minutes. Breathe to set your awareness of breath, to begin coordinating breath and movement, to perform your chosen type of breathing, and to immediately change your circulation and level of energy.

You can do breath priming either while standing with equal weight on both feet or sitting with a straight but relaxed spine. Your eyes can be open but unfocused, not blurred, just not focused upon any object, or closed and rolled slightly upward to focus upon your brow point where the eyebrows come together. The best hand position is to touch the first fingertip of each hand to the tip of the thumb. This takes advantage of the energy flows in your body called "meridians." Touching fingertips to thumbs keeps you calm and in a receptive state. Your whole body will now openly receive the new pattern of breathing that you give it.

Now pick either the complete deep breath or the breath of fire. Breathe steadily for one to three minutes. At the end of your breathing exercise, inhale deeply and suspend your breath for five seconds by lifting your chest a little, pulling in your chin while keeping your neck relaxed, and gently squeezing your lower pelvic region (navel point, sex organ, and anus). This is called "applying the root lock." Then relax your entire body.

For an extra energy boost, do the above breath priming exercise, but raise both arms up over your head, wrists straight and hands held as just described with the first fingertip of each hand touching the tip of the thumb. Fix an angle of sixty degrees between your arms held over your head and your body. Keep your elbows straight and arms up for the full length of your breath priming exercise. When you suspend your breath at the end of the exercise, keep your arms stretched upward. Relax them and let them drop when you finally exhale.

For extra relaxation and clearing away the day, use the complete deep breath. Focus at your brow point, and pay attention to a sound as well as to the flow of your breath. Pick either the subtle sound of the breath itself to focus upon, or repeat mentally the primal sounds SAAAAAT on the inhale and NAAAM on the exhale.

Awakener Exercises

Once you've done a breath priming exercise such as the one we've just taken you through, it's time to begin the series of sequentially repeated motions that makes up the main body of each awakener. The powerful effects of these sequential movements come from something called the "systemic training effect." This effect develops from sequentially performed motions that also possess balance, for example raising and lowering both arms. It turns out that when you move an arm or a leg on one side of your body, you automatically create stimulation in the limb on the other side of your body. Exercises that take advantage of this basic principle use the rhythmic stimulation of alternating movements back and forth between sides of the body to create a combined training effect that far exceeds the direct effect of simply moving a single limb. You can see this applied in martial arts, tai chi, yoga, and exercises designed for rehabilitation. The result becomes the creation of a balanced strength in the muscles.

Awakeners use something that goes beyond a warm-up stretch—holding a posture with a mindful breath. When we hold a posture, we don't stretch a muscle directly but rather stimulate the muscle indirectly by putting pressure on the organ area of the body that relates to the muscle. For instance, when you put pressure upon the navel and the lower intestine area by holding the right posture, you free up movement in the hamstring muscles. According to the applied kinesiologists, people who study muscle strength and motion, every muscle responds to the level of stimulation and the functioning of certain organs in the body. The hamstring muscles will contract and lose flexibility if the large intestines do not function well.

Here's some everyday proof that you're familiar with if you've ever gotten the flu. Let's say you can normally reach down and touch your toes in the morning. But try to reach down for your toes when you're getting sick, and you quickly find out that touching your toes is like a distant dream. You accomplish your usual stretch only with notable pains behind the knees.

A mechanical analogy for pressurizing one area of the body to affect another is to think of it like squeezing one end of a long, skinny balloon in order to get the other end to bulge. Holding a posture takes advantage of the reflex zones, points, and meridians that relate muscles, nerves, and glands throughout the body. The correct awakener will use a sequence of postures to release a flood of energy directed toward the muscle groups that you wish to increase in strength and flexibility.

There are some general guidelines to use when you practice the awakeners that go with the Breathwalks in the guide.

- The rhythmical motions of arms and legs in the awakeners begin and end smoothly with inhales and exhales.
- Hold your final posture for a moment and suspend your breath when you bring an awakener exercise to an end.
- Begin inhales at the start of a motion, not partway through the motion. Then the motion that you make gently drives your breath. Do not push your motions with the force of your breath. Let your breath relax and

become natural as it follows you. Make sure that your basic breathing pattern is to inhale by relaxing the abdomen, exhale as your navel goes in toward your upper body. Upper-chest breathing alone will be difficult and produce discomfort, tension, or dizziness. Become comfortable with good breathing as described in earlier chapters.

- Once you set the breathing pattern in an exercise, forget it and focus on the motion itself or on your point of concentration. Your breath is used to running automatically. Be aware of it. Once it is going right, let your breath energize you to support your other efforts.
- Always breathe through the nose, unless specifically instructed to use an alternative pathway.

Why Awakeners Work

You may wonder how awakeners can be better than traditional warm-up exercises. Most of us have been trained to think about the body in very mechanistic terms. If we think mechanically about warm-ups, they are to raise the core temperature of the body and flush the circulation to support the raised level of metabolic activity accompanying vigorous exercise. Stretches provide balance to the muscles that you will strengthen through your exercise efforts. Stretching those muscles first allows them to deepen their full range of motion and flexibility when you work at strengthening them. The goals of normal stretching warm-ups may be summarized as smoothly raising the systemic level of body activity, increasing flexibility, and reducing injury by keeping the body balanced.

Instead of thinking about your body with a mechanical metaphor where you increase flexibility by using out-side force upon it, think about it as a responsive community of organs, glands, and muscles. Now optimal flexibility and health come from increasing the communication and cooperation among the appropriate parts of the community and by stimulating local members directly. It makes sense to get a greater impact by using effective teams of community members rather than relying upon an isolated member.

Unlike warm-ups whose sole purpose relates to your muscles, awakeners emphasize the following areas that go beyond simple fitness for your muscles.

BREATH. You will use your breath as an integral part of al-most every awakener sequence. Breathing works as a tool for achieving maximum effect from all exercise.

STILLNESS. Some awakener exercises have you simply hold a posture for one to three minutes as you consciously breathe and direct your attention. Holding your posture takes advantage of your body's high level of connectedness. When you hold a posture, you create a pressure in a spe-cific area of your body. That pressure can stimulate your muscles to adjust; the pressure triggers a meridian to open and flow and to alert the body's innate intelligence to cor-rect the function and form in the pressurized area.

REPEATED MOTIONS. Many awakener exercises use a re-peated motion, such as swinging your arms or lifting your legs. These motions, coordinated with your breath, are done steadily for a specified interval. Rather than a stretch re-peated a few times or an exertion against resistance done a few times, many awakener movements are repeated sixty times a minute. The repeated small efforts within an awakener exercise have a large cumulative impact.

SEQUENCES. The awakener exercises are performed in sets, done in specific sequences. The exercise sequences create balance within your body and mind and emphasize particular desired effects. Stillness is blended with repeated movements to produce "synergies"—combined effects greater than those possible from either stillness or sequences performed alone.

ACTIVE ATTENTION. Attention means that you create a point of focus, either within or outside of your body. When you attend to something, the mere fact of your attention changes the thing that you focus upon.

Our bodies possess an intricate system of muscles, nerves, circulation, and glands—combined with an active mind. These all work together like a responsive web, not like a set of mechanical levers. We are responsive biological creatures that learn, adapt, and draw on an innate intelligence passed on through aeons of development. If we use those inner gifts, we can change in the blink of an eye and use exercise to gradually expand our awareness, health, and spirit.

Points to Remember

- Begin with breath priming. Breath priming involves taking a few conscious breaths to set up a flow of breathing from the vast store of breath energy that we possess within and around us.
- Perform all physical movement in the sequence that each awakener calls for. The correct sequential movements stimulate combined training effects that multiply the total impact of your exercise many times over.
- Synchronize breathing to motion. Then each motion that you make gently drives your breath, which releases inner energy and thoroughly awakens the whole body-mind.

6 ALIGN—Breathwalk Step #2

WE CAN, AND OFTEN DO, WALK WITH OUR
mind in one place and our body in the other.
Most of us just aren't trained to be fully present in our bodies while we exercise. This second Breathwalk step—alignment—assures a
conscious link between our mind and body.
When we align ourselves for conscious, mindful walking, we are prepared to learn, to let in
new thoughts and feelings. It is simple and
natural and adds entire dimensions to the pleasures of walking and meditation.

Without the awareness that alignment
can bring, we tend to experience walking in
utilitarian terms. It is just a way to get us from

point A to point B. Walking when we are aligned and aware, on the other hand, is about much more than just getting there. Walking can awaken our sense of simple joy and contentment in the moment. It gives us a "time-out" from our problems and lets solutions find their way to us. All our activities seem lighter if we can open up to the sense of contented joy that is wrapped inside each moment. Then even a brief walk can refresh our spirits. Walking reminds us that we are more than machines, greater than our jobs, freer than our fate, and born to happiness in our essence and spirit.

Start Slow

Walking contains quite a range of speeds. Just as horses have different gaits, some fast and some slow, so do we. When we walk we go through different paces—strolling, normal walking, striding, and speed walking.

Strolling. Speed range: 1.5–2.75 mph. Average speed is about 30 minutes to the mile, or 2 mph.
Normal Walking. Speed range: 2.75–3.5 mph. Average speed is about 20 minutes to the mile, or 3 mph.

Normal Walking. Speed range: 2.75–3.5 mph. Average speed is about 20 minutes to the mile, or 3 mph.

Striding. Speed range: 3.5–4.2 mph. Average speed is about 15 minutes to the mile, or 4 mph.

Speed Walking. Speed range: 4.2–4.8 mph. Average speed is about 13 minutes to the mile, or 4.6 mph.

Race Walking. Speed range: 4.8–6 mph. Average speed is about 11 minutes to the mile, or 5.5 mph.

Walking can benefit us even when we do it at a very slow pace. The slowest pace is a stroll. It is leisurely and free, usually uneven in pace and characterized by frequent halts to take in a view, sniff a fragrance, converse with a friend. A stroll is mild exercise that invites you to sense the enchantment of your environment, senses, and friendships. Strolling is the place to begin as you master the variety in the art of Breathwalk.

If you're starting to rehabilitate a tired and out-of-shape body, or a distraught mind, strolling can begin to elevate and transform you without injury, risk, or extreme effort. We've witnessed this firsthand in the people we train in Breathwalk. Those who could not walk a full mile in thirty minutes when they began practicing Breathwalk have reached fifteen-minute miles and now walk three or more miles daily after nine months. They have lost weight and gained a new measure of the possibilities of life—as well as dramatically lowered their measures on a number of health risk factors. All by strolling!

Many walkers try to increase their speed because they want to achieve higher burn rates to use up calories. They know that caloric expenditure increases rapidly—nonlinearly in fact—with speeds above 4.5 mph. However, we encourage Breathwalkers to use a slightly slower pace to get the widest range of walking benefits. Caloric expenditure, which is simply weight moved over time against an incline, does not equate directly to body conditioning. Body conditioning involves communication among all the tissues of the body, glandular responsiveness, emotional balance, and aerobic capacity. Paces slower than speed walking actually work better for stimulating the full range of communication among all levels of our body and mind. As you will learn in the next chapter, in the third step of Breathwalk we vitalize by alternating intervals of conscious breathing with regular walking. This accelerates many of the benefits of walking so you get them at much lower speeds. And the experience of a slower speed becomes filled with energy and pleasures you thought could come only with greater effort and speed.

When we teach people how to walk properly as part of learning Breathwalk, we begin with a stroll or slow normal walk and then gradually pick up the pace to a speed comfortable for the walker. In our training we call this a "pace-up," and we'd like to briefly explain how this works before discussing the second step of the Breathwalk—align. Begin by walking normally, creating a gentle, systematic warm-up. Then gradually increase your walking pace to a speed that you feel comfortable continuing for the next fifteen minutes or so. This provides us with the chance to do a "systems check." Pacing up sets a steady motion to our walk, establishes our body rhythm, and directs our attention to this exercise and away from the thousands of involvements and distractions that we have pulling at us. Pacing up should take one to three minutes. By the end of the pace-up you should be walking somewhere between 1.5 and 6 miles per hour. It should be a speed that you can comfortably hold at a steady pace and rhythm.

Don't just charge right into a brisk walk. Pace up gradually to warm up both body and mind. This one- to three-minute period turns out to be an important prelude to your whole Breathwalk experience. While you pace yourself up to speed, you also check on your walking style and consciously improve your posture and walking form to be efficient and even elegant.

Conscious Alignment

We all walk without giving much thought to it. If we had to think about each muscle we use and determine the complex interplay among our muscles to walk, we probably could not manage to walk at all. Some things are best done by reflex. In fact, people who concentrate too much on every movement, trying to reach perfection, end up walking in a stiff, mechanical manner. That does not mean that a periodic focus on how we walk will not pay dividends. It's very easy to unconsciously fall into bad walking habits. Those habits may become hard to break, lead to a physical problem, or reduce the potential pleasures of walking.

A good approach to improve your walking style is to start where you are. First, walk as you normally do. As you walk, run through a mental checklist (see page 113) for each area of your walking form. Then, add small corrections to what you already do. Great athletes and dancers improve in this manner. Golfers and swimmers use it to improve their strokes. Use your instinctual motion and refine your walk gradually. Remember, your body has an innate intelligence gained over aeons of time that readies you to act and move smoothly. Trust that inner sense. Finally, add conscious instructions to incrementally develop an improved form, closer to the ideal.

Align your awareness and body form to put elegance in your walk and vitality in your flow of energy. As you pace up to a normal walking speed and stride, try bringing your conscious attention to your walking form. Ask yourself, "Am I walking correctly?" and do a systems check. How are your feet, ankles, and knees moving? Do you feel any unusual sensations or pains that you need to pay attention to? Continue scanning until you have checked the condition of all your bodily movements, both small and large. "Scan" your whole body and make any corrections necessary to achieving a perfect walking form. When we teach Breathwalk, we call this practice a "body scan." If you experience difficulty "seeing" yourself in this manner, try doing what we have done for some students. Have a friend videotape you walking, so that you can review your form and visualize your movements.

As you check the condition of your body part by part, also survey your inner mood. How do you feel about the day ahead? How would you like your feelings to change? Which feelings do you want to invoke and intensify? Pay attention to the feel of the whole body, and note where your attention lingers or fixates. We hold attention just as we hold tension in different areas of our body. By noting consciously where we hold attention in our body, we give ourselves permission to redistribute that attention and release the tension.

To align fully, you need to do two things. First, run through the basic checklist for good posture and form, like a pilot running through a preflight checkoff list. Second, add attention consciously, like an artist surveying his or her creation—noticing every feeling and nuance that the image and shape of our body gives us. We will cover these basic mechanics first, then use the art of mindfulness in the body scan to complete this step two of the Breathwalk.

Gradually your mindful attention during a thorough body scan will produce a sense of presence. Body and mind come together in the present. Your mind will synchronize its attention with your movements and with your conscious intention to do this activity now. You will become alert, aligned, and fully present.

From hundreds of meditation, exercise, and walking workshops, we have learned that these two things—good posture and alert presence—maximize the pleasure and power of walking. Adding good mechanics and the art of conscious attention to walking triggers a cascade of benefits: elevated moods, easy walking, no injuries, spontaneous grace in movements, physical conditioning, fun, and motivation for life.

Getting your posture correct and aligned allows you to dwell on the other sensations and pleasures of walking. Checking posture lets you recognize the condition of your body before you exercise and tells you how well your body is working when you begin walking. Attaining good posture releases accumulated tensions and encourages natural healing as you walk.

Good posture results from three factors: physics, emotional attitude, and learning. By physics, we mean the mechanical laws that balance the forces among muscles, gravity, and the human skeletal structure. Just to stand and walk on two legs requires a lot of balanced forces. For example, the motion of the pelvis while walking involves a tilt and rotation. The motion of the torso appears as a combination of swing and torque that exquisitely counterbalances the motion of our pelvis and legs. These opposing forces must be applied in exactly the right rhythm and strength to permit us to both balance and move forward—to walk at all.

Beyond complex mechanics and laws of biophysics, posture also involves our attitudes. Negative attitudes produce poor posture. How we feel about ourselves will show up like a shadow in our outer posture. Think better about yourself, and stand tall! Posture is not about looking right for other people. It's about aligning your body for optimal ease and effectiveness of movement and breathing. It's about the inner grace that reveals itself in elegant outer form and style.

Posture is maintained through our emotional attitudes. We express our moods, our inner emotional states, through posture—the essence of dance and the performing arts. Try to feel happy with your body all slumped over and your chest caved in, and you will get the idea. Or try to feel sad with your arms uplifted wide, head up, and chest expanded. These postures don't match the inner attitude of these feelings. Either the posture or the mood will have to give way.

Here's what actually happens. Emotional attitude changes your chemistry, and chemistry shapes your posture. So when you take on a posture, it is an act of attitude. When you choose to keep a certain emotion within you, it reflects itself in your posture and your movements while walking. Conversely, consciously directing your posture into the correct form automatically triggers chemical changes that uplift your emotions and change your mood state. This means that you can fix those negative emotions by shaping up your physical posture—an important clue as to why Breathwalk can use physical motion to alter or enrich your emotions. Posture and mood are connected by a two-way street.

Posture requires learning because the laws of physics demand a wide range of coordinated muscular movements to accomplish the single goal of walking erect. Because of the range of motions that permit walking, we can often recognize a unique signature in a friend's walking style.

Breathwalk

Posture works as a coach for all of the muscles engaged in walking. If you think about standing straight or lifting your chest, you automatically start to use all the other muscles you need for walking more effectively. You need to pay attention only to a single cue—the position of your body—not all the millions of microlevel muscular movements. That's why a checklist of main postural cues works to give proper shape and flow to the whole body. Good posture is much more than just standing straight. It is about attitude and movements that flow smoothly.

Checklist for Good Posture and Form

How can you know that you've got your posture right?

START WITH YOUR FEET. Check the angle of your feet when your heels strike the ground. The angle should be about forty degrees, a little less than halfway up toward vertical.

CHECK THE ANGLE BETWEEN THE TOP OF YOUR FEET AND YOUR LEGS. It should be near a right angle, ninety degrees. Some people have learned to slap their feet down almost flat. This takes the cushion out of the arch support mechanism. Others have learned a style that "flips" the front of the foot upward. This style lacks focus upon the heel, locking the ankle. A good heel strike places the force through the heel itself and extends the leg out straight. When you get the foot angles right, the momentum of your weight actually carries you forward with little effort on your part.

Here's the proper sequence. Roll your weight from heel to toe by striking the heel lightly but firmly. Next, shift your weight forward through the arch as the foot rolls along the bottom of the outer toes. Finally, shift your weight across the ball of the foot and the big toe as you actively push off from the middle of the foot.

STRETCH YOUR LOWER BACK AND STRAIGHTEN YOUR TORSO. Good walking posture helps alleviate many back problems and strengthens the abdominal muscles. Poor walkers slouch a little and lean forward. The best posture comes about when you imagine your spine stretching upward and the lower, arching part of your back getting more of a curve in it. Picture in your mind's eye such a thing. Imagine a vertical line from the center of the top of your head down to the ground. Lengthen your lower spine. Now notice that when you allow your torso to lean beyond that line, you bring your weight to bear on the lower back muscles, straining them. When you align your spine with that imaginary vertical line, your lower back and abdominal muscles delicately balance your whole torso with a perfectly matched, but light, set of counterforces.

OBSERVE YOUR CHEST. Lift your chest up slightly, as if you are being pulled upward and slightly forward by an invisible hook attached to the upper part of your breastbone. Picture it in your mind's eye. Let your shoulders relax and drop back. Don't squeeze your shoulder blades together. That would make you lose balance, sway, and strut. You need motion in your arms and ribs, so relax your shoulder blades. Feel that your chest is open and moves with your breathing to lead you forward.

PERCH YOUR HEAD UP, CENTERED AND BALANCED. When your head gets off balance, you throw off the rest of your body trying to compensate. When you align your head, your shoulders, chest, and spine will tend to follow. To set your head correctly, make sure that you have lifted your chest slightly first; then let your eyes look toward the horizon, keeping your head level and chin pulled in slightly, but not down. When you do this, the center of the torso and the solar plexus tend to relax. Your abdominal muscles naturally pull in and tighten. Feel the areas at the base of the back of your skull, the occipital bones. This juncture between the base of the skull and the spine should feel relaxed. Now when you walk you can actually feel a gentle pulse or responsiveness there. If this area relaxes, it sends out a reflex that helps the lower part of the spine—the sacrum—move freely. Check that the muscles of your throat and neck are relaxed as well. If you put your head down and forward, these muscles will tense up.

If you walk as though you are being led by your head, you will pull forward of the imaginary vertical line. Then your shoulders will automatically roll forward and compress in your chest. Your breathing will be interfered with, creating problems for your lower back. As you can see, one improper thing leads to another, until you place yourself into severe distress.

CHECK AND RELEASE YOUR SHOULDERS, HIPS, AND KNEES. Posture is maintained by the smooth swing and counterswing of arms and legs. Scan your shoulders and arms, then your hips and legs, and finally your knees. Notice your shoulders. Make sure that they feel loose and level, directly in line with both your ears and your hips. Now feel the weight of your arms. Let their weight release, and sense that release falling all the way to your fingertips. Don't hold the tension and sense of the weight of your arms at your shoulders. Send that weight along the full length of your arms as they swing naturally. Let your arms swing smoothly at your shoulders like pendulums. No pushing from the chest or back area, even when walking at higher speeds or when pumping the arms in a fast stride. Imagine that pendulum-like weights descend to your hands and that your arms swing freely. Let your natural rhythm keep all of this in synch, in perfect rhythm and movement.

SHIFT YOUR ATTENTION TO YOUR HIPS AND LEGS. Let the weight of your legs "release" and extend along their entire length to your feet. Feel that the natural swing of your legs and their weight open a space in your hip joint, so that the movement becomes flexible and frictionless. Notice the motion of your hips. They rotate and undulate in wavelike cycles. Your pelvis naturally rotates about four or five degrees to either side of the vertical gravity line of your spine. The pelvis moves downward on the opposite side to the supporting leg, cushioning your body. All this translates into some pretty complex motion affecting the triangular-appearing sacrum, the lowest part of your spine. It's the area at and just above your tailbone. It wiggles a bit from side to side with the rhythmic pelvic motion, and it tucks a bit under and then back again with the movements of your breath and the contractions of your diaphragm.

FINALLY, NOTICE THE MOTION OF YOUR KNEES. Your knees should not wobble from side to side as you walk. This joint is the most complex in your entire body, held in place only by muscles rather than a strong skeletal fit. That's why the human knee is so injury prone in sports. Walking is kind to the knee, unlike running, which stresses it with too much weight and impact. Scan the motion of your knees. They should not be "skulking." Many beginners doing a brisk walk bend the knee at full extension and do a "Groucho" slide to increase speed. This interferes with the pelvic motion and also makes your feet slap the ground with a flat foot sensation rather than roll from heel to toe. Your walk now becomes jerky, and you increase the strain to your knees. When you are walking, your knees should feel steady.

Once you've scanned your entire physical mechanism while in motion, here's a good way to finish up. Walk slowly and feel the smooth flow of energy throughout your body—the pleasure of motion, the rhythmical waves of walking that run from head to foot. Now shift attention to your breathing. Listen for the primal sounds of your own breathing or to music you may enjoy while walking for a few moments.

The first time you do a complete body scan of your walking posture in motion, it should take you between three and ten minutes. With practice you will soon be able to do an effective scan in only one to three minutes as you begin walking. Taking time to visualize all of the results and to feel each area of your body functioning smoothly will begin to place each right motion into your muscular memory. Your motions will become automatic, effective, and enjoyable.

Mental Alignment

As you scan your body and pace up to a brisk walk, the eye of your conscious mind focuses on one area of movement and then another until you finally lock into muscular memory the complete settings for smooth, efficient movement. But where do you locate your mind after you've established your well-tuned posture? There is always a mental posture, an alignment for your mind, as well as for your physical body. Centering your mind on a single alignment point eliminates stray thoughts and helps you focus upon your main activity.

You can consciously choose a location for your mind, a point of projection and mental viewpoint, after you've set your posture. You've already aligned the physical parts of your body, why not align your mind as well? This idea may seem strange at first. But we literally hold our mind and project it from different locations whether we are aware of it or not. In the martial arts, for instance, you learn to set your focus near your center of gravity, at the level of your navel point. Another common alignment point is near the heart center at the middle of your chest. The world feels different from here rather than from the navel area. The third common center is the brow point, the forehead just above the nose.

Most of us instinctually pick a place around or in the body to walk from like a center or fulcrum for our actions. We do it without even realizing that we're doing it. Sometimes we move that point hither and thither over many places as our thoughts wander. That movement is dictated by a complex mix of emotions, training, and physical condition. But remember, you can select and direct a point of mental projection. This is almost always done for top performance in dance, sports, martial arts—and for a good Breathwalk.

Experiment with these three focus centers as a final touch to setting your mental posture. Imagine a shining thread of laser light projected from your body, originating at the navel, heart, or brow center that you choose. Imagine it stretching out ahead of you parallel to the ground. As you walk, follow the thread of light as if it pulls you or goes right through you. Experience walking from the navel, then shift to the heart and then to the brow point. You can experience a distinct difference as you project from each center. The thread of light focused through the navel feels solid, steady, powerful, and earthy. Through the heart it feels open, spacious, receptive, and optimistic. Projecting from the brow gives a sensation of confidence, lightness, flying, and detachment. Once you pick a center to walk from, set it and let go. Now you're just walking and letting your body without effort hold that center with the thread of light.

Body Image and Successful Change

The brain holds an image—a map of your entire body's shape and functions—all in 3-D space. It remembers this image and can respond to anything involving your body by updating the information in its map from sensory data. How do we know that this 3-D body mapping actually takes place? Studies show that when people lose significant weight and are then asked to draw accurate pictures of themselves, they usually draw themselves as much heavier than they really are. Their internal image has not yet been updated, and they respond with actions and emotions that do not align with their actual condition. This results in clumsy feelings, awkward movements, and lowered motivation, all because actual change has not yet been acknowledged.

Part of living in the now involves the process of continually updating the mapping of your own body, so that inner reality conforms to outer sensory information about you. Then confusion diminishes and calmness reigns. There is a kind of mindfulness that arises when you achieve the presence that we have been describing. Learning becomes totally experiential, not conceptual, as when you dwell in the head. Learning can now happen over your whole body, cell by cell. You can command the cells of your body to learn a new image that corresponds to the one you visualize. It is the supreme example of the power of your own body's innate intelligence at work. Using this step to align your body, combined with the changes created by Breathwalk breathing patterns, you can update the inner image of your body and mood clearly and rapidly.

The science behind how this happens is pretty complex, but what it all means in practical terms is that the mindfulness achieved in so vividly scanning the body arouses systems within the brain. Scanning the body, especially when the body undergoes motion as in pacing up to a brisk walk, triggers brain areas such as the cerebellum, sensory cortex, insula, hippocampus and their associated brain systems to reprogram your inner body image and the feelings that go with it.

This practice has many practical uses. When you wish to change your weight or alter a long-term depression, for instance, you can first connect and communicate with the cells that constantly reproduce or hold your old experience. Visualizing your body holding a proper form while moving puts you into a rapid relearning state. It brings the inner image you were holding up to your desired state so that you can physically change quickly and effectively.

Without this tangible process to create a new inner image, your efforts to change are often derailed. You create a thought without the power of your desire, or one part of you tries to change without the cooperation of the rest of you. You slip and fade back into the old pattern very quickly because the core cellular memory and learning have not changed. You communicate with the conscious part of your mind, but you don't reprogram the unconscious. The key to all permanent change in these areas is to connect to the unconscious and to cellular memories of the old pattern. Then break those patterns and consciously create a new energy and template for future actions. Practice the new pattern until it happens without your even thinking about it.

Weight loss and other life-improving processes begin with inner body image. Reprogram your body image and you can begin to change your weight and your dominant mood.

After you awaken, take a few minutes to align. Bringing body and mind together in the present is enjoyable, healing, and easy to do. It prepares you to reap the benefits and magnify the impact of the third step of the Breathwalk—vitalize.

Points to Remember

- Pace up gradually to your normal walking speed.
- Alignment comes as you scan your body and mind during the pacing up. It perfects walking posture and mental presence.
- Consciously directing your posture into the correct form automatically triggers chemical changes that uplift your emotions and change your mood state.

7

VITALIZE—Breathwalk Step #3

YOU HAVE NOW REACHED THE HEART OF Breathwalk—the place where breath and walking, pattern and rhythm, all come together. We need to focus on several details in order to do this step correctly and enjoy the full range of its effects. It is like learning the keyboard and scales before we get absorbed into the natural flow and beauty of a sonata. After we learn the fingering for the music, we can forget it and shift our attention to the melody and impact of the harmonies. We will focus on putting our steps and breath together, on the ratios and patterns we use, and on alternating intervals of walking with a breathing pattern and walking in a relaxed stride. Once you learn these details, you can easily shift to the big picture to focus on the energized feelings and clear mind that come with a Breathwalk.

The combination of instinctual rhythms and breathing makes it effortless to do. With a little precision we synchronize the breath and our steps with specific ratios of time for the inhale and exhale done in intervals of concentration and relaxation. Though we need to be precise, the rhythms are easy and organic. Read the details in this chapter carefully and then let your feet and your natural rhythms bring it all together as you walk.

Three Elements for Vitality
- Breathing and walking timed together
- Breathing patterns, which combine a breath ratio and breath type
- Vitality intervals—walking with and without the breathing patterns

Breathing and Walking Timed Together

Breathwalk at its very simplest means putting breathing patterns and walking together into a carefully and beautifully timed single, synchronized movement. It is walking harmonized with breathing. Each step that you take in your walk propels a measured portion of breath, and each portion of breath commands movement. Walking and breathing become intertwined. Almost automatically your steps will follow the commands of your rhythmical breathing, and your breathing will trigger from your steps.

To get a sense of how breath and movement combine in distinct ways, just think about how horses move. Their movements have been studied in great detail with video and computer analysis to find any useful advantage in creating champion racehorses. When you watch a well-trained racehorse move, you can witness elegance in motion. That elegance shows how only certain ratios of breath and step fit together and are stable.

Watch a horse begin with a slow walk and gradually increase its speed. It has many complex interlocking systems that let it walk or run. It does not increase the speed of its legs in a continuous manner. Instead it has only certain fixed patterns it can maintain. A well-trained horse finds those patterns immediately and matches them to the speed it wants to go. It begins with a slow walk. Then it goes to a trot. Then to a canter. Then it breaks into a full-out gallop. In a trot diagonal pairs of legs move together. In a full gallop all four legs are off the ground during each stride with a three-beat rhythm.

If you look even more closely, you will discover the horse's breathing locks into the movement of the legs in certain fixed patterns. Each gait—stroll, trot, canter, and gallop—has a corresponding breath pattern as well as leg movement that uses energy efficiently and that the horse can maintain without error or injury. Each walking or running gait requires a breathing rhythm, and each rhythm sets a horse's gait. Our breath and walking rhythms also have certain combinations that work best. When we use them we walk smoothly and get great results for moderate efforts.

It doesn't take a great, strenuous push to create a major impact in our body or mind. The pulse of our synchronized breathing and the waves of effort in the vitality intervals use a pendulum principle to build the energy. Just think of a swing. Each cycle of the swing goes a little higher and more energetic. To increase the height of the swing, we push it gently and precisely at the still point of its arc. If we push sooner, we fight its momentum, and later our push loses some power. The same principle applies to synchronizing our walking motion and breathing pattern. Precise, gentle breaths nudge our energy, awareness, and total vitality higher as we walk.

As we continue to walk and consciously breathe together, we awaken and connect more and more areas of our body. Some areas may have been partially closed off from a free flow of energy and communication by habitual emotional patterns reflected in chronic or traumatic tension. Those areas need a gentle wake-up call to break out of their habitual posture. Then they can communicate and participate better with the rest of our body and mind. The steady pulsing of the breath frees those patterns. Once all the areas of our bodies start to respond and act together, learning, conditioning, and mood elevation all get magnified manyfold.

Breathing Patterns

Once we can walk and breathe in harmony, we want to add a conscious breathing pattern. A "breathing pattern" consists of two parts—breath ratio and breath type. You already know that breath ratio is merely the time you spend inhaling compared to exhaling. Some breathing patterns use equal time, others use unequal time. "Breath type" means complete, smooth breathing or segmented breathing. A breathing pattern is just ratio plus type.

Breath patterns added to walking let us target the effect we want—energy, mental clarity, mood control, connectedness, or a sense of spirit. Each pattern is part of the recipe for a particular effect of a Breathwalk program.

You can get the idea of breathing patterns very quickly by comparing these three examples. When you breathe normally, you are doing an equal ratio, smooth breathing pattern, quite automatically. When you do the basic 4/4 segmented breathing exercise from chapter 4, you consciously use an equal segmented breathing pattern four steps on the inhale and four steps on the exhale. A pattern we use in another Breathwalk, called the Hawk, uses an unequal ratio with segmented breathing. It is done with eight steps on the inhale and four steps on the exhale. That means that in an 8/4 segmented breathing pattern you take twice as long to inhale as to exhale since the pace of your steps stays even like the ticks of a clock. Each of these three examples is a type of breath, segmented or deep smooth breathing, and a ratio measured by the steps, either equal or unequal.

Since your steps act as a timer, it is easy to learn the different ratios. Just use your steps to measure your breath. The easiest way to maintain both ratio and frequency of the breath while walking is to measure the breath with your steps. The following diagram shows you two breathing patterns in a simple graph. You can see what is different and what is similar from the graphic.

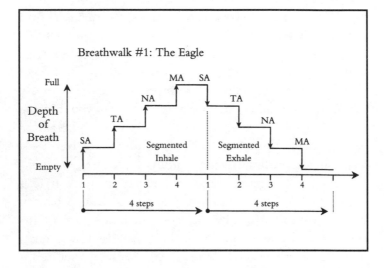

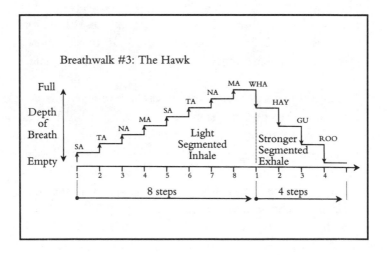

Each unique breathing pattern yields slightly different health and fitness effects, allowing you to zero in on precisely the areas of your body, mind, or mood you'd like to work on.

Breathwalk Breathing Patterns and Impacts		
Ratio	*Breath Type*	*General Impact*
4/4	Segmented Breath	clarity and energy
8/8	Segmented Breath	calmness, steady, endurance
8/4	Segmented Breath	energy, motivation, focus
4/8	Segmented Breath	slow down, cleanser, let go
4/4	Complete, Smooth	balanced, clear, and centered
8/8	Complete, Smooth	calmness, good digestion, fewer cravings, stress buster
8/4	Complete, Smooth	self-assurance, strong heart, great circulation, rejuvenation
4/8	Complete, Smooth	patience, let go old feelings and anger, lessen a habit, gain perspective
4/4/4 and 8/8/8	3-Part Complete	presence, awareness, regality

This table gives the essence of ten of the basic breathing patterns in Breathwalk. The ratio and type of breathing are listed along with some key words for their primary effects. When timed to your walking pace, they will allow you to change your energy levels and to direct your moods.

Students of Breathwalk often ask about the ratios used

in the Breathwalk patterns. They want to know if they can use other ratios. "Why do we just use these ratios?" We use only certain basic, even-numbered ratios in Breathwalk breathing patterns. These have been well tested for many generations and lead to stable, healthy, predictable states of mood, mind, and energy. Only certain combinations of breathing and movement create a powerful, stable, and predictable result. Just as a cake recipe needs a correct proportion of ingredients in order to rise and taste delicious, the elements in Breathwalk work when in correct proportion. The particular ratios we use in Breathwalk patterns come from centuries of experience in kundalini yoga and from the insights of modern research into biomechanics.

We can certainly imagine other ratios. We could try 3/15, or 7/9, or 11/6. The number of possible ratios is huge, but not all ratios are stable. Most are unstable and lead to erratic moods or uneven energy changes. This is very important. You can imagine spinning on ice skates in hundreds of ways, but only certain patterns keep you balanced without a spill. It works the same way with directed breathing in Breathwalk. Walking with the breath in ratios, spinning on skates, and racing a horse are all subject to the inherent laws of physics and physiology. The ratios we use in the Breathwalk patterns respect both and give you elegant and repeatable results. They match breath to the inner ratios in the design of your body.

During some of the research reported in later chapters, we found good mathematical models that showed why the "doubling" of the steps in the ratios optimized the use of breath and energy. Just try them yourself and trust the experience of people who have Breathwalked consistently for years. With these ratios, the patterns feel great and can be easily learned.

When our walking movement synchronizes in a Breathwalk pattern, we move, almost glide, as we vitalize. By using the different patterns in a Breathwalk program, we can select and refine the final state of mood, energy, and mind that we want.

Vitality Intervals

A vitality interval alternates a period of normal walking with a period of walking with a Breathwalk pattern. We may walk with a 4/4 segmented breath pattern for five minutes, then walk in a normal stride with relaxed breath for three minutes.

Many people have learned about training in intervals from aerobics. We are often asked, "Are intervals used the same way as they are in aerobic routines? Are there other reasons for using them in Breathwalk?" There are three fundamental reasons for using intervals: to maximize conditioning and training effect in the shortest time; to build stamina, reserve energy, and healing; and to increase emotional intelligence as it builds and stabilizes our state of mind and mood.

The first benefit we get from exercising in intervals comes from its direct physical effect. Intervals of exercise work better as a conditioning tool than does constant exercise. The body changes gradually. Practicing an exercise in timed intervals rather than in a single sustained burst of energy creates a wavelike, reinforcing contrast that accelerates learning. Body and mind are completely intertwined. Your mind learns change as much as you condition your body to change. Intervals increase the impact of your exercise within a shorter period of time.

The second benefit of intervals is that they build your stamina and reserve energy for the whole day. They increase your metabolic efficiency and make walking as effective as many more strenuous forms of exercise. Aerobics have trained us to look for a maximum heart rate zone to increase fitness. Though this is good for training, it is not the whole story. An aerobic benefit to your body *and* mind is one that improves the overall efficiency of your systems to utilize energy when you need it. Exercises that use a much slower heart rate can still provide this benefit, just more gradually.

It has been shown that even mild exercise for a few minutes at a time done a few times a day will accumulate great benefits for good health. The *Journal of the American Medical Association* reports in its August 26, 1999, issue that "brisk walking and vigorous exercise are associated with substantial and similar (to vigorous exercise) reductions in the incidence of coronary events among women." In an eight-year study of 72,488 women, they found that walking at three miles per hour (a mile in twenty minutes) for five hours a week reduced heart disease by 50 percent. Even one to three hours a week dropped our risk by 30 percent. The Associated Press coverage of this quotes Dr. Gerald Fletcher, spokesperson for the American Heart Association: "People seem to think 'exercise' means 'go for it.' Walking, especially brisk walking, is just as good as a rough game of soccer or hiking mountains, or going to a health club and lifting weights." Add to this all the additional benefits you get from Breathwalk, and walking should be at the top of our list for vitality and for aerobic impact.

For real stamina under stress, we need to look to more subtle measures. Another measure of vitality is not heart rate itself, but the "complexity" in the heart rate variability.

This is a technical measure that shows up as part of the signature of wellness we found in Breathwalk and discuss in chapter 11. This effect increases across the intervals and not just from one sustained effort.

The third benefit of doing vitality intervals is the impact on our mood and mind. It maximizes our emotional intelligence. Emotional intelligence is the ability to direct, select, and deal with feelings, moods, and states of mind. In Breathwalk we seek a *state*— not a level of effort. Achieving the right clarity and awareness in our minds is critical. Awareness and vitality reflect and guide our entire system, whereas a single measure like heartbeat or muscle tension can be too narrow. We can certainly notice our heartbeat going into aerobic levels as we Breathwalk, but there are other measures equally if not more important to vitality. If we shift the state of our mind and mood as well as our level of activity, then we release a cascade of positive, healthy changes throughout the body. Our athletic efforts are supported by our mental attitudes and moods.

As we do the intervals, our body and mind use the contrasts to quickly recognize and shift to a new state. We create a contrast between the breathing pattern and the relaxed pattern of walking. This contrast lets us get our emotional and mental bearings. We learn quickly how to find the state we are producing and how to find it later when we are not exercising. The exercise takes us into a place not just of increased heart rate, but of increased awareness. In that place we can drop old patterns and welcome in new perceptions of ourselves and others.

The vitality and whole body integration in Breathwalk can help even those with a high level of athletic ability. Chandra is a world-class runner and trained for the Boston Marathon by running over ninety miles a week. He also did some weight lifting. He wanted to learn yoga stretches from one of our students. His yoga teacher told him about Breathwalk. He was willing to try anything to get an edge in his training. Even a one-minute improvement is important at his level of performance. He added two half-hour Breathwalks and extra awakeners to his daily training. He found he could drop his weekly miles to fewer than sixty with no loss of training effect. He told us he could run with more fluidity and less stress. His time improved by over five minutes in the first three months of training.

All these details are the heart of Breathwalk. Like a heart, the intervals and patterns of Breathwalk let you pump vitality and awareness to every part of your body and mind. There is one more detail you can add that uses your fingers for wonderful effects.

Finger Magic

"Finger magic" is the use of special finger movements. The magic is the effects of vitality and healing from something so simple that it seems like sleight of hand. Finger magic works by tapping the fingertips with the thumb tips rhythmically in a sequence.

Tap your thumb tip on your index finger tip, then the middle finger tip, next the ring finger tip, and finally the tip of the little finger. Use about three to five pounds of pressure on each fingertip. Then go back to the index fingertip and begin again. This cycle of stimulation from first to fourth finger coordinated with the breath and the primal sound scales constitutes finger magic. Synchronize and time your finger contacts with your walking pace, breath, and primal sound rhythms.

The Three Impacts of Finger Magic
- Alerts the body to change
- Promotes whole brain communication
- Stimulates the meridians for optimal flow and balance

How Finger Magic Works

Our bodies contain memories and subconscious impressions etched in place during each moment of our lives. Incidents leave marks and sometimes scars that give shape to our character and personality. But life is constant change. When the body becomes fixed and nonresponsive to change, it has formed a shell, a mask, or armor. It is protecting itself. It clings to an old pattern or memory of tension. To let the old armor go, we have to alert the body to change. Then we can supply it with new energy and a new pattern. Finger magic helps the body become alert and ready to change.

Moving the fingers of both hands simultaneously seems to fire both sides of the motor cortex in our brains. It enhances the communication between the two sides of our brain. Look at any map of the brain's surface—the cortex. Different amounts of the area of the cortex are allotted to each area of the body. Surprisingly, the fingers and hands take up more area than the entire torso, although the torso is much larger. The hands are used for activities key to survival and for refined gestures. This capacity for complex articulation is what takes up more nerves and area in the cortex.

Fingers also have many reflex connections to other parts of the body and brain. Tapping each fingertip alerts the zones of the body and brain that connect through the finger we tap. The cycle of taps assists natural flows of energy in the body. Restrictions in that flow that come from past emotional or physical pains get overridden by rhythm and by repetition. When we shift the body's attention from the first fingertip to the last, it forgets quickly. When we go back to the first fingertip it is surprised, alerted again. This pulsing wave of alertness resets the body memory and helps to disperse the old patterns. Tensions are released.

Healers and yogis who have studied the body have discovered that it is full of meridians—channels of energy flow. They are partly electromagnetic, partly biochemical, and partly subtle. Several major meridians end or begin in the fingertips. By tapping them as you breathe and walk, you allow the flow to adjust itself. One reason for its effectiveness is that the energy flowing in the meridians over the fingertips reverses its directions, relative to the body core, at the tips.

The sensitive centers in the fingertips are called "radiance points." They shine like brilliant flames in the aura. Touching them in rhythm brightens them and increases the exchange of energy that can be used for healing others with therapeutic touch or for healing yourself.

With these details in place, you can practice all the programs of Breathwalk. You can vitalize yourself. You can begin to focus on the experience of the beauty and power of rhythm and breath in your body, mind, and spirit.

Points to Remember

- The heart of Breathwalk is the patterns of synchronized breathing and walking done in vitality intervals.
- The power of the patterns comes from the use of ratio, breath type, and breath rate.
- A vitality interval is when you alternate between a consciously controlled breathing pattern and a relaxed breath with normal walking. It multiplies the impact of your efforts.
- Add finger magic to your walking intervals for healing and faster change.
- Walking, even as little as five hours a week, has been shown to cut heart risk by 50 percent. It is just as effective as intensive exercises like mountain hiking, soccer, or running and without the injury potentials.

8 BALANCE—Breathwalk Step #4

AFTER WE CREATE A CHANGE IN OUR ENergy, feelings, and general state of mind, it is time for balance—the fourth step in Breathwalk. The time it takes to reach a balance, one to three minutes, is very short. Its effect is to extend the benefits from the vitality intervals, the last step we did, for the rest of the day. We accomplish this by consciously shifting the quality of our attention as we open the senses and by doing a series of fluid exercises to stretch and maintain balance in the muscles.

Creating balance, even for a few minutes, makes the world fresh and prepares us to act with intelligence and awareness. Sometimes it can open the moment to reveal a timeless and sacred dimension. Even though we work hard to keep some balance in our lives, the demands from work, family, and our own goals fight against that balance. We can be creative and reach that external balance better if we regularly touch the state of internal balance within ourselves.

The habit of creating a feeling of balance is an act of generosity to ourselves. It is like learning to be a giver. The best way is to give a little every time you earn or receive something. It is the same with the practice of balance. Give yourself a taste of balance every day and your accomplishments and persona will be more balanced.

In each Breathwalk we reach a conscious balance between narrow and broad attention, effort and relaxation, inner and outer focus, and between this moment and our projection through time. We pace down from our stride in the vitality intervals as we change our focus and then stretch. We can feel our muscles, breath, and nerves return to a more typical range of activity as we walk regularly and slowly with our arms relaxed and in a normal swing. This is when we can put a seal on our renewed mental and emotional clarity that keeps it fresh and available in our body and mind.

Opening the Senses

The senses are the key to the balance step of Breathwalk. We all use sensory strategies to pay attention to one thing and not to another. Those strategies become habits. They help to make us effective in the things we do, but they also limit our flexibility. The Breathwalk patterns in the vitality intervals stimulate those habitual sensory strategies to change. During the intervals your attention is drawn inward, into breath and rhythm. Your attention and energy is focused within you. Now it is time to distribute that energy and redirect your attention. To distribute the attention you have broken free from old strategies, you need to switch your focus to a wide-angle, receptive scan of the environment and allow all of your senses to be fully open. That switch from a narrow internal focus to a broad external focus creates a balance and prepares you to sustain the gains of your Breathwalk.

Our attention directs our senses to be more open or closed, narrow or broad. We may think our senses are always opened fully. The reality is that attention is a limited and precious resource. We apportion our attention in a way that lets us sense and react quickly with the most accuracy. Whenever we make a concerted effort to do something, our sensory window narrows or widens to match the task. Sometimes to do one thing well—say, playing music or remembering a telephone number—we block out everything else. Perhaps you have seen people turn off the car radio when they start to navigate streets in an unfamiliar location. They turn off their attention in the ears so their eyes can see. It is a strategy to reroute and distribute limited resources for attention to the most important task of the moment. We all have sensory strategies that we use as we go through our daily activities, strategies that mix our senses in a patchwork design where each sensory channel is either opened or closed. This gives us a combination of senses, each with its own abilities, that together create a particular focus. With the right focus we use our senses in a skilled way.

That same pattern of sensory attention allows us to attach our feelings and experience to selected cues. We can focus on our legs as we exercise, and we will associate the feelings we get with what we pay attention to—our legs and tight muscles, for example. How we direct our attention after an experience determines how accessible that experience is. With a broader awareness we can connect the experience to more cues and to other experiences we have. As a general rule, we narrow our focus to get a task done. That is why the practice of holding our attention broadly open can be so relaxing. It is the balance to the narrowing. Simple mindful meditation practices use this fact. Relaxations with imagery that take our mind to imagine wonderful vistas also shift the scope and direction of our attention.

During the vitality intervals, we usually experience some of this alternation between narrow and wide attention to our senses. Most of our attention during the intervals tends to be inward and concentrated. The breathing patterns and listening to or repeating primal sounds pull our attention inward. That focus amplifies and consolidates the changes we are creating. In step two, as we align, our focus is also directed inward to the details of our walking form and movement. When we switch from synchronized breathing to a regular stride, we may broaden our focus as we attend more to our senses or to conversation. Still the dominant mode of attention is more inward and narrow because of the powerful changes and sensations we release with the Breathwalk patterns.

After the vitality intervals we need to create a balance. We need to consciously shift our attention for a few minutes and open all our senses to every feeling, sound, sight, and smell. Direct nothing; limit nothing; take in everything. Switch from a close-up view to a wide-angle view. At the same time let thoughts and feelings flow freely as well.

Breathwalk

An easy way to balance your energy and make this transition from the vitality intervals is to first look, or listen, to something that attracts you—a person, a tree, a building, an animal. As you pace down for one to three minutes, notice the details. Take them all in with all your senses. Then mentally move on to something else, and then something else again. Pay attention to every new sensation—vivid colors, unusual and familiar smells, the feelings of the space around. Locate yourself mentally in the here and now, in this moment, exactly where you are. Don't drift off or focus on a single thought or mental scene. Stay present and let all the thoughts and sensations pass freely through you.

Two things happen from this short balancing step. First, opening your focus allows the state we have produced with the Breathwalk patterns to last longer and the benefits that come with the state stabilize and become available to us throughout the day. No matter what combination of senses we need to use in the rest of our day's activities, a thread now connects us back to this peaceful, energized state of awareness. Second, we relax and become fully present in the moment. Without old thoughts and feelings blocking the experience of ourselves, we gain insight. With the senses open and filled with our immediate feelings, we become flexible and responsive to the messages of our body and mind. This improves both physical and mental health. The feeling of being awake and aware lets us enjoy every moment and acts as an antidote to stress and overload.

Triple Balance Stretch

The best cool-down after exercise includes some relaxing stretches—stretches that are active but targeted to one area, then another, until you are balanced. The lungs should be opened now and used to breathing in synchrony with your movements. That's what we do in the stretches. Without breathing a stretch can become a hitch or a cramp. With breathing a stretch frees and extends you, increases flexibility and feels great. When you exercise for thirty minutes or more, stretching becomes very healthful to do.

These stretches flex three main areas of your body: the upper back, neck, and shoulders; the torso, ribs, and mid-back; and the hips, calves, and legs, including the hamstring and quadriceps muscles. We will stretch each area in turn with a cycle of short, natural moves that we call the "triple balance stretch."

The triple balance stretch consists of three movement sequences that each relax, stretch, and distribute your energy in a major area of your body.

1. "Salute the Sky" clears your shoulders and upper back.
2. "Spread Your Wings" clears the torso and mid-back.
3. "Salute the Earth" clears the legs, sciatic, and hips.

Salute the Sky

1. Stand straight with legs together, arms relaxed along your sides. Inhale as you stretch your arms up over your head and join your palms together. Now hold your breath and hug your arms against your ears for 1–2 seconds. Then exhale fully as you let your arms back down.

2. Inhale as you lift both shoulders straight up. Hold for 1 second. Exhale fully as you let them down. Hold your breath out for 1 second as you let the weight of your arms at your sides pull your shoulders back down.

3. Inhale deeply as you raise your arms forward and up in a large arc over your head. Hold for 1 second and stretch toward the sky. Now exhale completely as you complete the circle by moving your arms over your head, down in back, and returning to your sides. Hold your breath out for 1 second, and let the weight of your arms stretch down while you keep your spine straight and chest slightly lifted.

4. Grasp opposite shoulders. Inhale deeply and tilt your head up about 45 degrees, or as is comfortable. Exhale and tilt the chin forward onto the collarbone. Hold your breath out for 1 second as you lift up your chest, pull in your belly, and squeeze your shoulders. Now inhale and straighten up, relaxing your grip.

Spread Your Wings

1. Stand straight, with your palms together in the center of your chest (prayer pose). Inhale deeply and hold for 1 second. Exhale as you swing your right arm out to the side and back. Turn your torso and head in the direction of your right arm as it swings back. Keep your other hand poised at the center of your chest, fingers pointing up. Hold your right arm in the extended back position for 1 second. Then inhale back to the center, both hands now again in the prayer position.

2. Repeat the same sequence with your left arm: exhale as you swing it back, turning your head and torso in its direction; inhale as you return to the center. Hold 1 second.

3. Then exhale as you swing both arms back, keeping your wrists bent and fingers pointing up, the head and torso facing forward. Hold at full extension for 1 second. Then inhale back to the center.

4. Repeat this full sequence 3–5 times.

Salute the Earth

1. Stand straight with your legs spread comfortably apart, arms held in front of you and parallel to the ground with the palms facing up. Interlace your fingers, palms together, and press the fingertips over the knuckles—this is called "hammerlock." Inhale deeply as you raise your arms over your head. Stretch and hold for 1 second. Then exhale smoothly, bend forward at the waist as you swing the hammerlock forward and down through your legs. Hold down and breathe out for 1 second. Inhale back up. Hold. Exhale completely as you bend down and swing the hammerlock over your right foot. Hold for 1 second. Inhale back up to the center over your head.

2. Repeat these motions, but now over your left foot.

3. Now exhale as you let the hammerlock go and return your arms to a parallel position to the ground and in front of you.

4. Repeat this full sequence 3–5 times.

5. Bend forward and make a triangle of your feet, hands, and buttocks. Your hands are flat on the ground and your heels are off the ground at a comfortable height. Relax your neck completely. Now inhale slowly, then exhale and hold your breath out for 1 second as you press your heels down toward the ground. Now inhale and release the pressure and let the heels rise back up. Repeat this 3 times. Then gradually stand up, inhale as you reach up, and then relax.

The triple balance stretch distributes energy and relaxes you. It counters any tendency to "bunch up" your energy or your tension in one area. It also gets the body to "remember" itself, to act as a whole. Using the breath as you move triggers a flush and reset of the lubricants between connective tissue fibers, the fascia. Your body's connective tissues are held together by collagen, a tough protein used throughout the body. Under wear and tear, the connective tissues accumulate calcium and adhesions that lessen their stabilizing and structural functions. The increased blood, oxygen, and lubricant flow that comes to these areas after exercise and a good stretch keeps them supple, reduces any postexercise pains, and relaxes the body. This gets to the source of where body inflexibility seems to develop—not in the muscles themselves, but in the connective tissues. Stretch for a few minutes and enjoy hours of flexibility and balance.

Points to Remember

- Balance follows vitality intervals in a Breathwalk.
- We create balance by opening our senses, shifting the focus of our attention, and doing a few fluid movements to stretch.
- The effects of this step are to make the benefits we created in the Breathwalk patterns more available through the whole day and to place us fully in the moment, aware, awake, and fully alive.

9

INTEGRATE—Breathwalk Step #5

THE FINAL STEP OF A BREATHWALK IS TO integrate. Once we have done this, we are ready to engage the world and ourselves anew. Our body is stimulated and energized. Our mind is clear and without conflict. Our spirit is welcomed and connected with. When we are integrated we become aware. We become consciously conscious and in complete synchrony with our mind, our sense of self, and our spirit. It is much more than basic alertness.

We use an Innerwalk to integrate. Innerwalks are a large collection of techniques that direct our mind and attention to create new sequences and patterns of thought. They guide the senses not just to open, but to break old patterns and to gain new ones. Once the mind is clear of blocks and connected to its inner resources, we can go confidently and with success from our Breathwalk to any path we have chosen.

An Innerwalk moves us along an inner path. It does not depend on our outer path. That inner path has a special feeling and quality to it. A student asked, "How long is the path to awareness and enlightenment? It seems far away, unreachable at times." Yogi Bhajan replied by spreading his hand wide open. He placed the tip of his little finger at the navel point and stretched the thumb tip upward until it touched the center of the chest the heart center. "It is just this far," he said.

The inner path of awareness requires us to move from the lower navel area that modulates impulse and instinct up to the heart center, where we are compassionate and aware of others as much as we are of ourselves. For invincible vitality and awareness, we need to travel that path. Along the way it combines all the power of the senses and passions into a balance that can express our spirit and our soul's capacity for depth and subtlety. If we make that inner journey, then every outer journey will be fruitful and give us the experience of our spirit. Wherever we go we will end with character and happiness. Innerwalks help us along that path to the heart center.

Doing an Innerwalk takes anywhere from one to fifteen minutes depending on the Innerwalk you choose and your purpose for doing it. You can do one while physically walking, pacing down to a stop, or sitting still in quiet contemplation. Each Innerwalk guides your mind in different ways. It may direct the images in your mind along the path you are walking, or internally through your body as you sit, or with imagination to new places somewhere in the universe. The real beauty of learning the Innerwalks is that they give us a way to insure good communication from our heart to our head and from our head to our heart.

An Innerwalk is as much an attitude as a technique. It's a kind of posture of the heart. It is where we meet each moment with innocence and openness as if it has never come before. A good Innerwalk moves us along the path to open our capacity to love and the power of our heart center. Some techniques work by increasing awareness and magnifying the senses. Some remove distractions and bring our focus into the present. Others remove hazards and pitfalls by clearing emotional blockages. When the path is clear and we awaken inside, we can reach the heart center and let it open wide.

It is easy to recognize when we have integrated our mind and emotions and opened the door to our heart center. There is a timeless moment of clarity. In that moment of clarity we feel present and alive. All our senses scintillate with stimulation and wonder. Our bodies feel vibrant; our minds become alert and open, the many voices from the battle of inner conflict now quiet. Here, in the stillness, we have become both alive and *more* than alive. We have become *aware* that we are fully alive and ready to live life. The heart center triggers spontaneous healing, and the body and mind can reorganize with the guidance and radiance of our spirit.

We can enter this place within ourselves spontaneously on a rural stroll, or passing a mountain vista—or even on swift dashes between buildings at work. The only real place we find this center is inside ourselves. When we integrate at the end of our Breathwalk:

Certainty conquers doubt,
Healing soothes distress,
Clarity replaces confusion,
A Flow comes in the midst of turbulence to show
the way, and
Radiance bursts out from within the darkest of
moods.

We know exactly where we are and with certainty what to do in any situation.

With this awareness, we can sense the entire range of our emotions. Not a single feeling is restricted or lost to us. Yet we find ourselves so peaceful and balanced that we do not feel the need to react to any of those feelings except the ones we choose to embrace. Spontaneity and a sense of freedom now dominate, rather than our past compulsions or impulsiveness. Keenly aware of our surroundings, we feel somehow deeply connected to them. Our sense of time changes. The moment seems timeless and hints of eternities. We find our simplest actions woven smoothly into the greater purpose of our lives.

The best of all true things is a true heart. Without truth there is no happiness, though you may try a million tricks.—Kabir (Sakhi, 64)

What follows will guide you with precise words and encourage you to try each technique for a practical experience of personal integration. Do not just read these pages, live them out. Learn with your whole body and mind, just as you wish to live with your whole body and mind. When you find something that triggers your interest, touches a need, or sparks your intuition, try it.

Five Innerwalks for Body,
Mind, and Spirit

Start to think about your senses as a pure gift, the gift of six senses—our primary five senses and a sixth sense. Call the sixth sense intuition. We all experience the world and ourselves through a blend of these six senses. Now it's a simple fact that by birth and genetics some senses for each of us appear stronger than others. You may, for instance, have an excellent "ear" for pitch and tone, or an "eye" for subtle shades of color. More important, we learn to favor certain senses over others. We use our senses to represent the world, to prepare ourselves for action in the world, and to limit those experiences that we do not like in the world and seek out those that we do like. Each of us develops our own sensory patterns based upon our experiences and learning. We may expand some senses and diminish others.

In this manner we form conscious and unconscious sensory habits—through natural inclinations and learning. Walking and breathing in harmony can break the automatic sensory patterns that we've programmed ourselves for—and thereby open all the senses for our pleasure and instruction. Breathwalk changes the settings for our senses by impacting the autonomic nervous system to let in new feelings and fresh information. You become vitally connected to the present, with your senses now wide open. You become alert, responsive, and alive to the moment.

Try each of these three Innerwalks and notice how they awaken you to expanded sensory experience.

Gathering Your Senses

We call this Innerwalk "Gathering Your Senses." Literally that is what you do. We experience things best when we gather all the sensory pieces into a luxurious and vivid whole. You can do this Innerwalk while physically walking. It can be done sitting down, but walking seems to work best. A good way to do this is to walk for a short while with your focus on one sense at a time. Then walk with all the senses open at once just before you end the walk.

To begin, walk with your hands open and relaxed. Curl your index finger in on one hand (or both), and start to pay attention to what you see. Then curl in your middle finger(s) and pay attention to what you hear—both the outer sounds and your own inner voices. Then curl in your ring finger(s) and pay attention to smells. Notice new smells; notice the absence of smells. Now curl your little finger(s) and notice tastes. We actually experience many nongastronomic tastes that reflect our emotions and our physical health. Last, curl your thumb(s) over to form a fist as you now sense all your feelings at once.

To end, spring open your fist(s) and become aware of everything around you and in the universe all at once. Let your senses scan and take in everything. Use your intuition to feel your next step and how this step connects you to the rest of the path, to the rest of your life and to the world. Finally, walk for a few minutes without concentrating at all; let your senses play freely, directed and stimulated by whatever strikes you on each step.

Sensory Bubble

This next Innerwalk is called the "Sensory Bubble." Instead of enumerating the senses, you imagine the surface of your skin expanding outward like a giant sensory bubble. The bubble surrounds you. It has an exquisitely sensitive surface. The best way to do this is to sit still in a meditative state. Let everything in—every sound, feeling, thought, smell, and taste. Become very still in the center of the bubble. Rest within your heart. Use the feeling and image of the bubble to sense things in all directions at once. One direction may seem more open or easy to feel than the others. That's fine. Sense that, too. Open that area up. Become totally transparent. Become subtle. Sensitive. Restrict nothing—even allow the feelings of tensions and contraction to come and go. Only the mind limits reality and the senses. Use your mind and its imagination to let the sensory bubble gradually expand for feet, yards, miles, hundreds of miles, light-years, to the unlimited.

Notice the flow of your own breath as one of those sensations. Feel your breath throughout the entire sensory bubble. With each breath reestablish your still point, your center. Let each inhale bring you to alertness, and on each exhale let go of what you sensed and how you held it. Feel, bless, and then release everything. As you extend the sensory bubble evenly in all directions and become increasingly still, you will sense one of the great pleasures of Innerwalking as you move bit by bit into the vastness of your heart center. Most people like to do this for three to five minutes. End it with a deep inhale. Suspend the breath for five to ten seconds, then exhale completely. Repeat this last breath three times and stretch the arms up.

Walking the Breath

This Innerwalk is called "Walking the Breath." It is longer and has a definite sequence to its steps. It is especially good for self-healing and for a deep relaxation that is very rejuvenating. It is a direct way to work on your light body, chakras, and meridians. We use it in several of the Breathwalk programs in the guide section of this book.

To begin, become aware of the flow of your breath. Just notice it and its qualities—slow, fast, smooth, full, or shallow. As you dwell upon these sensations, notice how the breath seems to fill the body; notice how breathing creates waves of motion throughout all parts of the body into each limb, each area, and even each cell. Think of the life-giving properties of the breath—the gift and pulse of life itself. Wherever it flows, there is movement, energy, and vitality. Build on this thought and feeling as you follow the flow of your own breath.

Feel that the breath is more than just oxygen. Think of it as a subtle radiance, energy, or source of life. As you breathe in, feel the sensations of the breath expanding throughout your body, in past the skin and circulating all around you. As you exhale, see it as a glow of light; hear its gentle sound surround you and project outwardly. Feel your breath leave you, and imagine that you now project light out into the universe. With the power of your mind, connect the tidal ebb and flow of your own breath to the universe—as if it is an ocean of energy flowing in and out of your physical body and in and out of your radiant breath-body.

Now imagine the sensation of your breath coming in through the crown of your head and traveling down your spine as you inhale. As you inhale, let that feeling fill your entire body, spreading out from the spine. When you reach a full inhalation, sense your body glowing, strong and radiant in all directions. As you exhale, guide your breath to gather and flow like a river of light along the spine, upward and forward to your brow point. Then let it continue to flow out into the universe as it goes from your brow point and down off the tip of the nose. Walk the breath this way for one or two minutes.

Now inhale slowly and "walk the breath" from the fingertips of your left hand along the arm to the center of your chest at the heart center. As you reach a full inhalation, feel the breath fill your whole torso and visualize it glowing intensely and comfortably with light within you. On the exhalation, walk the breath from your torso and let it flow down your arm and out the fingertips back to the universe. Walk the breath this way three or four times. Now switch and walk the breath from the other side—from the tips of your right hand up the arm to the heart center and then back down again. Do this three or four times as well.

Now focus the flow of breath on a walk starting from the left toes and sole of the foot, up the leg, and gathering at the navel point area in the lower abdomen. As the inhale becomes full, sense the breath glowing from the navel and filling the whole body with an intense healing light. As you begin to exhale let all discomfort and distress leave the body, flowing through the navel center, down the leg, and out the toes of the left foot back to the universe. Do this slowly and consciously three or four times. Now switch the walk to the other side—from the toes and sole of the right foot up along the leg, gathered at the navel center, and back down with the exhale.

Now focus and walk the breath along a path that starts

in both feet at once. As you take a slow, deep inhale, mentally guide the breath flow up along the legs and join them together at the navel center like two rivers mixing. As you complete the inhale, lead the breath from the navel area up the middle of the torso to the heart center. As the breath reaches a maximum, feel an intense radiance from the heart. So one deep inhale goes smoothly from the toes of both feet, to the navel area, and up the center to radiate from the heart center. As you exhale, project the breath from the heart center into the world. Imagine it like a great breath that clears your way, a radiance that spotlights your path and secures each step you will take. Repeat this entire pathway three or four times.

Now focus and walk the breath from both hands with a slow inhale, up along the arms and joining together at the heart center. As the breath becomes full, feel its pressure and glow fill the torso. As you begin to slowly exhale, walk the breath from the heart center back into the spine and upward through the neck and out through the crown of the head and back into the universe. Project it as if you could send a gust of wind all the way to the farthest stars. Release the breath with a sense of gratitude and with a trust that another will come. Repeat this Innerwalk three or four times.

Now inhale very slowly. Sense the entire vastness of the cosmos. Walk the breath through the crown of the head, down the neck, and along the spine. Imagine the breath flowing out into every cell of the body. Let each cell begin to shine, warm and radiant. When the breath is fully inhaled, feel the body bursting with light and energy. Feel the entire surface of the skin. Feel the skin in front, back, sides, top, and bottom all at once. Then as you very slowly exhale, imagine each pore of the skin as an outlet for the breath.

Imagine each pore sending out a beam of light—blue white light, a brilliant light such as you can see when an arc welder works or in a spectacular flash of lightning.

Extend that light from all pores at once for miles and miles as you exhale. Create a ripple in the cosmos with this breath. Then begin the inhale through the crown of the head again. Repeat this cycle as long as you like. Then bring your focus to the brow point or forehead. Suspend the breath in a meditative lightness for a minute or so. Then take a deep breath, hold briefly, exhale like a cannon shot through the mouth. Repeat it again. Stretch your arms up to the sky. Turn slowly left and right twice. And relax.

You are ready for anything! Once you have walked your breath through all these inner channels, you can walk any outer path with energy and success. There are many technical reasons and much thought behind this particular sequence. It has been used by thousands of students with consistently positive results. Remember to practice the visualizations and the sequences before you set out to do it. Then you will better remember each path that your breath will follow. When you do this as your final step in a Breathwalk, you will create a profound and memorable experience.

Play and Replay

We recommend this particular Innerwalk to revitalize yourself after long hours at work, to center yourself and be more present, and to conquer stress or break the boredom from an emotional rut.

To prepare yourself for this Innerwalk, take a few minutes during your pace-down to open all of your senses to the environment around you. Now sit somewhere comfortable and close your eyes. Roll your eyes up slightly, let a slight smile cross your face, and lift your cheeks and the corners of your eyes just a little.

Focus through the forehead as if you can mentally see a panoramic screen. On that screen watch a movie of the walk you just completed. Go back to the beginning of your walk—all the way back to the awakener and to the first steps of your pace-up. Replay the entire walk. Review it step by step, frame by frame, so to speak. Hear the sounds at each part of your Breathwalk; feel how your sensations changed in each area of your body along the walk. See all the scenery—the people and things along the path. Recall the scents and locate them along the path. Take enough time to replay the entire walk, ending up exactly where you now sit doing this replay.

Now, consciously notice something about the way that you just replayed the walk. Did you use all of your senses? Where did you experience the replay from? Did you put the mental recorder or camera in your body or outside, viewing from a distance? Did you view the replay through a narrow-angle or a wide-angle lens? Did you retrace your steps in a steady pace, or did you vary the pace for different parts of the walk? Become truly conscious of the replay that you just did as if you are a cinema critic. Observe the quality of the production, the choice of camera angles picked by the director, the use of sounds and inner commentary.

Replay the walk again. This time locate yourself behind your eyes. See things through your eyes. You will not see your whole body, now you are in it. Be sure that you do not raise your focus above or below your eyes. As you mentally walk, adjust the picture and widen the angle a bit.

Raise the brightness to a comfortable level. Pay attention to details you may have missed before. With each scene you encounter again along the path, add in the sounds. Let the sound strike you from all sides. Then add the body feelings, the sound of your own breath, and all the smells you encounter. Complete the entire journey until you are sitting right here where you started out—eyes rolled up slightly, a slight smile, sensing the flow of your own breath.

Now replay your walk again. This time locate your self inside an imaginary walking partner or inside your actual partner if someone walked with you. Now see your body walking. Notice the scenery pass by, looking ahead and sometimes looking over your body that walks next to you. This may seem a bit odd to you at first. It shifts your whole point of view and lets you take in information and feelings about how you look from another person's point of view. It breaks the pattern of your normal, straight-ahead focus. It lets in a range of new feelings. You may now notice things that you missed on your first replay.

Heed your feelings about the walk, your self, and your moods. Watch the miracle of breath at work. Appreciate your efforts and your transformations along the walk. Complete the journey by watching yourself sit inside your body and focus on the forehead. Then imagine that you go into the forehead and slip back inside your body sitting where you are. Stay with your new sensations as you notice the flow of your breath going in and out, slowly and calmly.

Replay the walk one more time. This time locate yourself at a distance from your body. Take a very wide view so that you have to move only a small amount to keep seeing large segments of your walk. As you watch, you stay very relaxed. Alert all your senses. Extend your senses to notice distant sounds and sounds that you may have missed as you concentrated on walking or conversing. Move the cinema along quickly and smoothly until you reach the point where you sit. Move your mental camera completely around yourself. See your calm posture and gentle concentration from every angle. Now mentally float over the top of your head and slip down into your body. Return to your normal position inside your body and looking through your eyes. Let everything you felt and learned sit with you as you simply notice the flow of the breath for a moment.

Finally, be aware here and now with all your senses. Notice how the replay has changed your awareness. Take note of how it feels to have such rich and well-detailed information and feelings about yourself and about what you just did. Remember any lessons, ideas, or feelings that seem useful to you. Imagine keeping this state of openness and alertness with you through the rest of the day. Imagine walking from this spot, keeping all your senses open and flexible. Imagine each hour in the remaining day. Feel that you walk through each of those hours with strength, vitality, and full presence. Imagine how good it will feel at the end of the day looking back on the path you have walked. See how good it is to be ready to notice and act upon every opportunity. When you feel ready, take three complete deep breaths. Then hold your breath briefly, exhale, and relax.

The Whole Brain Cinema

This Innerwalk uses a classical eye-scanning pattern. It will help make all your thinking resources available to you. When you master it, it will give you ways to increase your range of emotional choices and insight about how your thoughts impact your body and mind. It is also a great aid to creative pursuits and to generating a feeling of wholeness and connectedness.

Begin with your eyes relaxed, eyelids closed and eyes looking straight ahead. Replay your walk rapidly from the beginning to the end. Now imagine yourself walking along your path from the beginning. Position yourself mentally inside your body, and invite in all the thoughts, feelings, and senses you have experienced. As you walk along the mental path, repeat the following sequence of eye movements, coordinated with your breath. Do the sequence as many times as you need to cover the entire pathway of your walk. However, if you have not become used to regulating your breath, do not exceed ten minutes in this exercise. If you find yourself feeling motion sickness or becoming disoriented, you might try doing the sequence more slowly or using a different Innerwalk, although many people who have suffered from motion sensitivity say that this exercise has actually removed their symptoms. Experiment for yourself.

Here's the eye movement sequence coordinated to breath: Look down the tip of your nose with your eyelids one-tenth of the way open. Inhale very slowly into a complete deep breath. Exhale completely as you pull in your navel point. Then roll your eyes up and focus upon the brow point at the top, or base, of your nose. Keep the eyelids nearly closed. Next inhale again slowly, sensing each movement of your breath. Exhale very slowly. Then inhale deeply and suspend the breath. As you keep your breath suspended, move your eyes two times along each axis—up and down, left and right, diagonal up right and left down, diagonal up left and right down. Complete one wide circle around to the left and one around to the right. Exhale completely. Then inhale deeply and suspend your breath again. As you keep your breath suspended, move the eyes spontaneously in all directions.

Once you have become used to the eye movements and the breathing, imagine walking along the path that you took for your Breathwalk. When you combine the eye movements and breath patterns with the mental replay, you may notice that particular feelings leap into focus and get processed.

To complete the whole brain cinema exercise, repeat the pattern one last time once you have arrived at the journey's end. As you do this final repetition of the eye movements synchronized with your breath, focus upon whatever activity, problems, or feelings you sense as most important to you. Then inhale deeply, stretch your arms up toward the sky, open your eyes, and look toward the horizon. Slowly exhale, let your arms down, and relax.

Whenever you need to engage your whole brain to understand your experiences, to solve problems, and to break through impasses or bring all your habits in line with your new goals or vision, use the whole brain cinema during your Innerwalk.

Points to Remember

- Integrate is the key word for this final step of the Breathwalk. We want to integrate our senses, the sequences of our senses and feelings, and the state of mind and energy we have created with the Breathwalk patterns. Integrated, the benefits of the state will build over time, go with you as you work and play, and seed the deeper opening to your spirit as the mind is cleared and commanded.

- The way we integrate our state at the end of a Breathwalk is with an Innerwalk. Innerwalks are a large collection of techniques that direct your senses and attention to adjust the flow of mind. They can use the vitality and awareness from Breathwalk to clear mental blocks, awaken emotional and spiritual resources, and heal and enhance creativity.

- Three basic Innerwalks are Gathering Your Senses, Sensory Bubble, and Walking the Breath. These are used with dozens of Breathwalk programs listed in the guide to enrich and expand your experience and command of your mind as well as body.

10 Using Primal Sounds with Breathwalk

WALKING AND SOUND RHYTHMS GO TO-
gether powerfully and naturally with the
breath patterns you have learned. They add a
further dimension to Breathwalk because of
their power to align the flow of thoughts
with the experiences of the moment.
Through sound we can create a calm center
within, by changing the flow of our inner
chatter—our self-talk. The most common use
of primal sounds during Breathwalk is
through the repetition of four basic sounds in
an elementary scale. We call them "primal
sound scales." We repeat them either mentally
or out loud, depending on our purpose. The

use of sound, mentally or out loud, leads to a spectacular increase in the intensity of our awareness and our ability to direct our actions, select our moods, and heal ourselves.

Primal Sounds

Primal sounds are the most basic building blocks that construct words. They make up the simplest primal speech units, the smallest units of speech distinguishing one utterance from another. Linguists call them "phonemes." They underlie words as atoms underlie matter and rock underlies earth. They serve as bedrock for all natural language.

This is why they are so universal. You may hear them as sounds like SA, TA, NA, MA, PA, GA, DA, NEE, SO, RE, RA, HAY, GU, WHA, NEE, KA, ROO, and others. Like atoms, they can be strung together to make molecules of sound—regular words that we use in daily language. PA, for example, can mean "father" in some languages but means "get" in another. The sounds gain a meaning, a semantic association with other words. Another way of using them is even more universal. Each fundamental sound has a quality that induces a kind of energetic gesture within us, just as hearing the pure note of a flute or a well-struck guitar chord evokes certain feelings. We understand that energy regardless of the larger piece of music it is embedded in, regardless of the language someone may give to it. In the same way, each primal sound, when listened to intently, is a gesture of energy, a pattern of qualities within itself.

The sound SA is open. It flies off the tip of the tongue and vibrates from the central cavity of the mouth. It feels open and vast. In the East, the musicians and yogis who studied the subtleties of these sounds assigned a meaning based on these qualities rather than on its use as a separate word in some language. SA, as a quality of energy, feels like and means totality, cosmos, or open to the universe. If you just repeat that sound slowly and steadily for a few minutes, you indeed feel vast, relaxed, and open. Compare that with the sound TA. It is pressured, shot from behind the teeth, and pressurizes an area at the top of the mouth toward the front. It feels energetic, directed, and intentional. As a primal sound it means life, energy to be and move, or the universe condensed to this living moment of existence. SA and TA are distinct and almost polarities of each other.

Primal sounds are used according to their energy, the pattern they produce when you say them rather than meanings in one language like English, German, Hindi, or Mandarin. They are in this sense words before language. They belong to no one, and we all use them.

Primal Sound Scales

A sequence of primal sounds can be used together as a primal sound scale. Primal sound scales have a special and universal character. They are a kind of do re mi for our awareness and state of mind. When we repeat these scales, the pattern of the scale activates our brain and evokes different states according to the patterns in the sounds. There is also a reflex code that connects the movements of the tongue with the neural patterns in the brain. There are eighty-four reflex points on the upper palate of the mouth. They are distributed along the base of the teeth and in two rows along the central fissure of the upper palate. As our tongue moves and repeats primal sounds, the pattern sends a code to the hypothalamus at the base of the brain that alters us, opens the senses, and directs the flow of our impulses and thoughts.

This powerful mechanism means we can repeat very basic patterns of primal sounds and have profound effects that refine and open our awareness. Through centuries of experimentation and use, certain scales were found to be especially effective, stable, and universal in their positive effects.

How to Use Primal Sound Scales

To use primal sounds in a Breathwalk experience, begin with the simple scale SA, TA, NA, MA. Four sounds, each a basic unit, each with its own quality and effect on our feelings, brain, and internal self-talk. As you do a Breathwalk pattern, begin to mentally repeat this scale to yourself, timed to your breath segments and your pace. Do not try to consciously block out the background chatter of your own busy thoughts; simply concentrate upon repeating the primal sound scale.

Primal sounds will create moments of true inner silence. Soon you will find that all the mental chatter ceases or moves into the background, far away. Your body, mind, and spirit will all come together with strengthened unity and presence.

Guidelines for Using Primal Sounds

1. Use primal sounds—root sounds such as SA and TA.
2. Use the two basic well-tested primal sound scales: SA, TA, NA, MA and WHA, HAY, GU, ROO.

There are more scales, but these two are fundamental and have effects complementary to each
other.

3. Use a simple monotone or three-tone melody.
4. Do the sounds silently or in a whisper, according to
   the instructions in the programs.
5. Coordinate primal sounds with your breath and
   with your steps during Breathwalk.
6. Concentrate effortlessly on the sounds to synchronize with them, rather than trying to block out
   other sensations or thoughts.

Two different melodies are used in repeating the primal sound scales internally or externally. The first is a three-
tone melody. To use the three-tone melody, let the second
and third sounds descend a note in tone from the first and
then raise the fourth sound up one note. Here it is in musical notation.

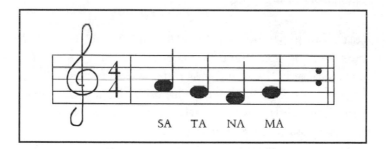

This elementary sequence with the final raised note at
the end creates a small novelty, a surprise, in an otherwise
regular cycle. The novelty alerts areas of your brain that deal
with executive attention function, memory, and under-
standing. This prepares you to learn, to accept new information from your feelings and senses. As you repeat it, it

goes into the background of your mind and is with you as you do other things. Your subconscious picks up the sounds and rhythm.

The second melody that you can use is a simple monotone. For this to be maximally effective, increase the attention you pay to the sound of your own breath along with the primal sounds, so that you create a beat accented by each step. This becomes very meditative and relaxing.

Primal Sounds and Your Inner Stories

The use of primal sounds helps us create positive internal states by interrupting our stream of self-talk and by facilitating our ability to edit our internal stories. Self-talk is all the phrases we say to ourselves, the questions we ask, consciously and unconsciously. They are the phrases and statements we weave together into a coherent story about ourselves and the world.

Our self-talk and our story are the primary ways we create our experience of the world and ourselves. We ask ourselves questions and make statements, even when we are not aware of it. "Do I like this? Is this what I want? Will this be fun or boring? Is this amount fair? Will this really make me healthier? Is this really who I am?" Those statements link us to our feelings, motivations, and beliefs. They are the difference between just thinking about something intellectually and being able to act on it.

To create the real and enduring changes that we want, we need a way to quiet the inner talk that does not support our intention and our awareness. Instead we need to use words that create and support a story, an inner narrative that is meaningful and effective for making the desired changes.

The steps from primal sounds, to words, to language, to metaphors, and to an inner story form a ladder from the most basic expression of sound to the normal awareness we all live with. Primal sounds work from the bottom up. Using them opens the way to change all the way up.

We build internal stories—stories we tell others and ourselves. With them we attempt to make sense out of the world and out of our feelings. Without such a story we would be overwhelmed with senseless information and with the anxieties that arise when things don't make sense. Stories help us form a model for how things are connected, what causes what, and what to do to get a desired result. They give us an internal reference point amid a flood of thoughts, feelings, and possibilities.

Stories can be hard to change because the brain is not unified. One area tends to give our dominant story and rationalization; other areas are less verbal and have stories full of feelings, not words. We lose control of those. We need to name things to use all the editing power inherent in our language structures. That the brain acts like a modular collection of many parts may explain the constant mental chatter that most of us experience. It may also explain why the stories we tell about ourselves often become divorced from our real emotions and potentials.

It's no wonder that we have so many inner conflicts and often block ourselves from acting with commitment and integrity. Without handling this tendency for warring stories within us, we develop extremes in our personality. The wonder is that we are not split more than we already are. Attaining unity, integrity, and consistency within us is quite an accomplishment. With the pressures of life, information overload, and speed of change, we need to do something consciously to maintain our center and sense of awareness. Here is where primal sounds come into play.

Once we form our internal story, we live our life through the lens of that story. If we want a great life, a fulfilling life, a life filled with love, challenge, spirit, and success, then we had better have a story inside ourselves that can lead us to that.

Lester Luborsky and colleagues at the University of Pennsylvania queried many patients involved in therapy about their stories. Dr. Luborsky had each person tell stories from many situations and time periods in their lives. After studying the results, the researchers discovered that people construct a central story for their life that encodes predominant conflicts or concerns. The concerns can involve family relationships, efforts in the world, or even intellectual struggles. But the same story and its supporting metaphors arose repeatedly like a texture throughout the person's experience. As patients were judged healthier and fully functional, the stories were more varied, less stereotyped, and the patient had gained some choices over how to tell the story.

The problem is that we form partial stories, good for one moment and not another, then forget to change the story. We become attached to a favorite story regardless of evidence to the contrary. Some stories are healing and functional, others are incomplete, fragmented, or downright dangerous. Over time our inner story gathers and carries with it limiting beliefs, outdated information, and rationalizations that deter us from taking the actions that we want. Guise and manipulation replace direct action and the power of innocence. We even use self-deception and lose track of who and what we have become. It becomes a real accomplishment to cultivate our words and inner story to represent consistently our values and purposes with our whole mind, brain, and feelings supporting them. The power of a story and our ability to make one is one of our great human advantages. We need to be able to modify our storyline to adapt it to new learning, circumstances, and our stage of maturity.

Most of us are aware of at least some of our stories. We can become aware of and edit our own story. We can "rewrite" our inner stories to be worth living and to be beneficial to others around us by using primal sounds as we walk to open our imagination, loosen the grip of words and phrases that anchor us to the past and to old behaviors, and to get our mind out of any small box we happen to be trapped in. It is up to us. We can fill our inner story with virtues such as compassion, or courage, or invincibility, or innocence, that inspire and help us be authentically who we are.

By using basic words in patterns, we can develop and activate our brain's ability to learn, understand, and perceive. We can actually awaken different brain areas through the words we use and the emotional charge that we put behind them.

Each phrase in the inner talk we repeat to ourselves acts like an anchor to hold us near certain feelings and beliefs. Mostly, if we notice the inner talk, we try to overcome it by saying something else louder. We repeat an affirmation or a denial with increasing intensity. This can interrupt the thoughts, but only briefly. It is like hearing a song you don't like on the radio and trying to sing loudly over it. If you succeed, you also create a lot of noise as well as discomfort for any friend nearby. A better strategy with the radio is to switch to a different channel. As the channel changes, so does the kind of music and the flow of thoughts that come through it. Without all the yelling, you can also hear your new song clearly.

That is how primal sounds work. Rather than an affirmation that overpowers your internal phrases, you change the frequency by using a basic melody of primal sounds. They are not whole words or long phrases, so they do not fight anything. They shift your attention and let the old phrases, repeated rationalizations, and internal tapes go. Then your mind will begin to give you new thoughts to support what you want to focus on and feel.

Primal sounds draw the many disparate parts of our mind into a working team. Rhythmical words act like an attractor for the many rivers of thought and feeling that come from the unconscious parts of our mind.

Primal sounds are a key to conquering our jumpy minds. Even when we find a line from a poem or a scripture that can still our mind temporarily, part of its potency comes from the beat and pattern of the primal sounds that make up the words and the phrases. Using primal sounds directly lets our mind focus its power beyond the flow of thoughts that compete for its attention.

The school of narrative therapists has moved close to recognizing the power we have to change our inner stories. They have had the insight that to speak is to shape and re-shape the neural connections in our brain. A pattern of speech, the sequence of primal sounds, and the structure of a good parable allow us to change habits and moods that have persisted for years or even for our entire life. In India the yogis called this art Naad Vidya—to know and heal through sensitivity to sound and story. By consciously using our words and sound, we can train our brain to act as a whole and lessen our internal conflicts.

This means that primal sounds work as the perfect neurostimulators to activate and connect many areas of our brain. This lets us create a new story and new vision. It is a deep source of creativity. Each single primal sound stimulates a unique response from a complex network in our brain. A simple primal sound scale works with the brain areas like a chord played on a piano that simultaneously engages a number of strings and sympathetically vibrates still more.

By adding primal sound scales to the synchronized breathing in a Breathwalk, we combine the emotional and physical energy we generate in the walk to the power of the sounds to free our minds, edit our outdated inner stories, and expand the horizons of our creativity and spirit.

Points to Remember

- Primal sounds are made up of basic units of sound called "phonemes."
- We most commonly use two scales of primal sounds with Breathwalks: SA, TA, NA, MA and WHA, HAY, GU, ROO. These two scales complement each other in effect and quality of energy.
- Primal sounds act as atoms of sound that can loosen the grip of our old or inappropriate inner stories, lessen conflict among our many parts, and clear out old stories stored in our subconscious.

---

11 The Science Behind Breathwalk

BREATHWALK HAS THE POWER TO CHANGE the basic rhythms of the body at system and cellular levels to produce an overall signature of wellness. When we look at what happens with the instruments and tools of modern research, we get a glimpse of some of the underlying biological processes that create the impact and benefits of Breathwalk. We have examined, with the help of professional researchers, the effects of Breathwalk in five fundamental areas important to our health and well-being—heart rhythm, visual focus, muscle balance, brain activity patterns, and moods.

We were excited to see that the initial research efforts into Breathwalk show that there is a rich area for further exploration. And we have seen some profound effects, as well as a way to begin to measure and track them. On a personal level we can all feel the vitality from a Breathwalk, and we can also sense the feeling of flow and power in our bodies. The change in our mental clarity and the acuity of our vision is immediate and tangible, and we can feel the more subtle impact on our spirit. But having conducted research into the benefits of Breathwalk, we think it is fascinating to be able to read that signature of wellness everywhere we look with precise instruments. It will allow us to understand and classify the many effects of different Breathwalk patterns and apply them to specific needs. Intuition and science can join together to map the ways to a healthier, happier life filled with passion and spirit.

Heart Rhythm

There are powerful and rapid effects of Breathwalk on the cardiovascular system, and practitioners report great increases in vitality and disease resistance. We decided to ask researchers for help to probe into the possible mechanisms behind these effects by participating in research on this matter at the Mind/Body Medical Institute and with labs at Beth Israel Deaconess Medical Center and Massachusetts General Hospital in Boston. The research confirms that there are special patterns in our heart rhythm and in our walking gait that do in fact develop as we do a Breathwalk. A similar pattern develops when we do certain breathing patterns and meditative exercises in the awakeners. These patterns seem to begin as we enter a special state of well-ness.

The preliminary results counter the common medical belief that meditation and breath exercises can produce only a physiological signature of reduced variability and di-minished complexity (increased periodicity) in the heart rhythm. In other words, a simple regular rhythm as we might get in a calm relaxation does not capture all the characteristics that we can produce during a meditative exercise like Breathwalk.

A leading researcher in nonlinear medicine, Dr. Ary Goldberger, offers this idea in *Perspectives in Biology and Medicine* (summer 1997). Dr. Goldberger writes, "As a general principle, disease states are marked by less complex dynamics than healthy states. Indeed, this decomplexification of systems with disease may be a defining feature of pathology. . . . Healthy systems are organized in such a way that they display (1) scale invariance and (2) long-range order." In layman's terms, when we are living vital lives many of our internal rhythms are "complexified" so that our organs, hormones, sensory systems, and brain can adapt to the unpredictable world we live in. Both random and extremely regular physiological signals are a sign of the system responding to some form of stress in a pathological way. The patterns we see generated and enhanced by Breathwalk and its conscious breathing patterns are exactly those of vitality and wellness in a healthy person.

One of the experiments worked like this. We first had volunteers walk and recorded their normal heart condition. Then we had them do a vigorous Breathwalk and monitored those results. As the volunteers did Breathwalking, their heart patterns changed substantially, suggesting the possibility of a distinctive signature of wellness. We could find a pattern that measured how much vitality and wellness the subjects had. Some of the same heart rate patterns were also produced during the active meditative exercises in the awakeners included in this book. The observed changes included a strong central frequency in the respiration and gait driven by the breath. The heart rhythm also locked into synchrony with them. The breath acted like a master key to synchronize several of the body's systems.

The patterns in heart rate variability showed features we are still exploring that look "fractal-like." They are complex and appear similar in form whether you look at them over three minutes or three hours. This self-similarity across various time scales allows healthy adaptation. It also seems to let the more regular rhythms of the heart, lungs, and legs work together without being rigid. Strong regular rhythms joined with the complex and nonlinear patterns allow for both smooth collaboration among parts and flexible responses. When your health breaks down—say, from congestive heart failure—the physiological signals like heart rate variation become either random or rigidly periodic. When the signal shows the fractal-like structure, it is not random and not a single periodic wave. Its complexity is a signal of health that shows a lot of communication and feedback from many parts of the body.

What happens to us experientially and physically when we enter into this state? When you do a Breathwalk, the pattern of your heartbeat changes in a special way. Just as doing aerobics creates a recognizable high-rate heartbeat pattern, so too does Breathwalk generate a distinct signature in the heartbeat. The aerobics heartbeat pattern results in a training effect that increases the body's ability to handle oxygen. The Breathwalk pattern shows the heartbeat running through a wide range of frequencies in a very short time period, promoting biologic flexibility. Biologic flexibility in turn has an important bearing upon overall wellness, because it reflects our ability to gain resilience and rebound under stressful situations. As the following example shows, using Breathwalk to get your body in rhythm can have profound immediate effects.

A participant at the Anthony Robbins Life Mastery University in Hawaii told us, "I had a very bad sinus problem. I was coughing a lot. I felt very bad and emotionally upset. Then I started to do this Breathwalking and it calmed me down, amazingly so, like within ten minutes. It gave me a lot of power. I've been doing it every day now and it's incredible."

If aerobic exercise resembles the pure power of a single frequency emanating from a strong radio station, then Breathwalk looks like the many frequencies mixed into complex and richly textured patterns. One is a tone, the other melody, chords, and harmonies. It is like comparing loud noise to sophisticated music. Breathwalk stimulates resiliency, rebound capacity, refinement, range, and flexibility—all adding up to awareness. And awareness adds another dimension to vitality that goes beyond aerobics and beyond the merely physical. The same patterns that give us a signature of wellness in the heart rate show up in our brain when we refine our ability to listen to music or improve any of our perceptual skills. Doing things that produce this signature of wellness improves our conditioning and our mind at the same time.

Visual Focus

Many of us have never even seen a recording of our own heart rhythm, and most of us are not scientists, so it can be a little hard to relate our practical experience to all the precise internal changes we've just mentioned. We have noticed directly and experientially, however, that the quality of our own vision—how clearly we see things—drastically improves in those who Breathwalk. First-time Breathwalkers frequently report that an amazing clarity comes over their vision; everything becomes more vivid. Depth of field, clarity of detail, and visual acuity all increase. People report experiences of delight as they seem to flow through an intensified sensation of three-dimensional space—an extended sensitivity of the body. You may personally experience this change for yourself just by Breathwalking. Listen to the experiences of these people.

> The world looks different now—immediate, clear, and alive. I have an amazing sense of visual clarity, and I feel as though I am flowing through three-dimensional space, ever so gracefully. Am I really seeing things differently?
> —A first-time Breathwalker

> I had an interesting sort of aliveness behind my eyes. It's like it wakes up your head. It makes you feel totally connected with everything below and above. And it comes with a certain feeling of tranquillity and energy! I recommend it to anyone who wants to feel good.
> —Ellen Bradley

The effects of Breathwalking on vision were strong and consistent enough that we thought we should be able to capture some data that would start to show us how people were really "seeing things differently." The improvements we noticed, besides being pleasurable, seemed to be very useful in coping with information overload. The ability to focus, to let go, to see things in different ways—our cognitive flexibility—is as critical to making good decisions as it is to enjoying art. We turned to an MIT colleague. His specialty is aeronautical engineering, but he has a knack for anything experimental. And Amrit just happened to have access to a computerized instrument that measures eye movements and pupil size using reflected laser light. When someone sits in a special chair and views some object, the machine sends out a small, harmless laser beam toward one eye. As the eye moves about to capture the object's appearance, the laser beam is reflected back to different locations that can be recorded in the computer and plotted on a graph as an eye movement pattern.

We had several volunteers look at two pictures while sitting in the special chair, and we recorded their eye movements as they focused on each picture. Then we had them do one of two different Breathwalk patterns. The first pattern, called the Blissful Eagle, is for energy, stimulation, and the ability to act with decisive clarity. It uses a 4/4 segmented breath. The second pattern, called the Dove, stimulates receptivity and emotional capacity. It uses an 8/8 segmented breath. After they had performed these Breathwalks, we put our volunteers back in the chair for a second time, once more recording their eye movement patterns. When volunteers did the Blissful Eagle Breathwalk, their ability to focus upon the central object in a scene increased dramatically; unnecessary eye movement dropped to a minimum. On the other hand, the Dove produced a wider-ranging eye movement that permitted volunteers to capture the full emotional content of the scene, but again with increased economy of movement. This is the image the volunteers saw:

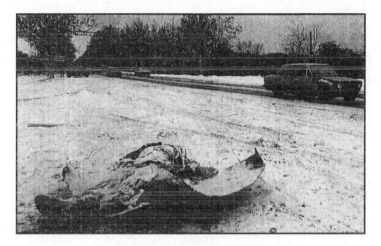

And this is the effect each Breathwalk had:

First Ten Seconds Looking at Fractal Before Dove Breathwalk

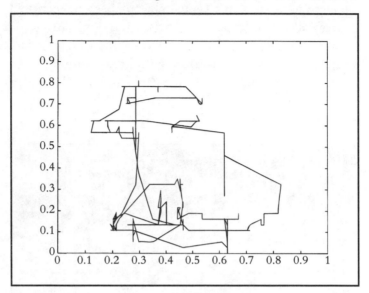

First Ten Seconds Looking at Fractal After Dove Breathwalk

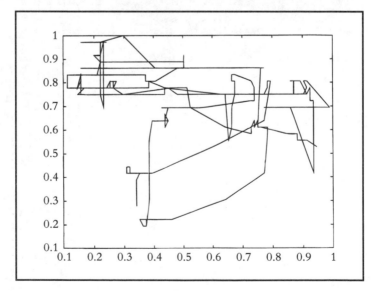

First Ten Seconds Looking at War Scene Before Blissful Eagle Breathwalk

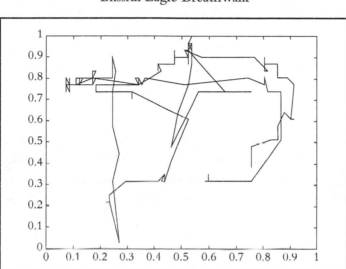

First Ten Seconds Looking at War Scene After Blissful Eagle Breathwalk

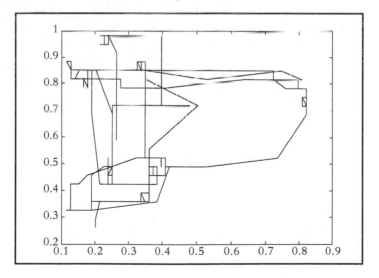

Clearly, then, Breathwalk can positively affect our vision. Most of our capacity to see and derive pleasure from the world lies dormant within us. We live in a comfort zone, rather than a zone of full vitality and awareness, and Breathwalk helps us open up our potential to enjoy and make choices in our perception. Seeing becomes more pleasurable, vision sharpens, and new aesthetic dimensions appear.

Both tradition and science tell us that we have all learned patterns of tension and attention—ways of attending to things around us. We often follow our habit of attention rather than shifting our attention spontaneously with what we see. The result is tension between our habitual pattern of attention and the pull of our immediate senses. This tug-of-war can consume a lot of energy, slow down our reactions, and lead to misperception. The tension we hold within us also constricts our vision. This means that we consume tremendous amounts of energy burned up in inner tension itself. For example, when you drive in a new area of the city and you are tense from rushing, work, or perhaps an argument, you will frequently fail to see the most obvious road signs, landmarks, and parking solutions. Tension in fact makes our vision work like a flashlight in a large, dark room: we can scan only one very small area at a time.

Breathwalk has the power to release us from the patterns of inner tension and free up our vision. Science has confirmed what yogic tradition has long taught. The pathway between our eyes and our brain works as a two-way street. Our eyes respond with pleasure to arousal and to certain ordered patterns. That arousal can come from either the exterior environment or from inside the nervous system. The brain influences what you can see, and what you can see influences the brain. By stimulating our brain in Breathwalk, we can gain insight in our inner world and in our visions of the outer world. We open the way for stronger and richer connections.

Muscle Balance

Look at how we regard one another. What do we actually see when we look at another person? We invariably record something called a first impression. That impression, right or wrong, lasts and affects everything else we see.

The first impression we make is usually a visual one. It is the fastest—faster than sound, as fast nearly as the speed of light. It comes way before any touch. It comes before we have a chance to have conversation. Even a slight change in our posture and movement can change how we feel and how others feel about us. The way we move and carry ourselves determines the visual imprint that we make. Clothes and accessories are important but secondary.

Breathwalk can make us look better. It changes how we carry ourselves and therefore the impact of our first impression on others. We can find one key to this effect in a quote from Dr. George Goodheart, founder of the widely used healing system called applied kinesiology. In his professional training manuals Dr. Goodheart says, "People look the way they do for a variety of reasons—hereditary, occupation, etc. But the primary pattern of body structure [and hence appearance] rests upon a balance or imbalance in the postural muscles of the body. 'Depressed' people generally show it in their posture, as do 'stiff-necked' and 'stuck-up' individuals. People look the way they do because the normal muscles contract and pull, and the weakened muscles allow them to."

When muscles weaken, become imbalanced, or suddenly collapse under some load, it signifies a problem in the body. We all have a deep instinct to look at posture and movement, because these two things give us an instant readout on a person's cumulative state of health. We become suspicious of odd movements and limps because of our instinctively sensed connection of them to physical and emotional states of disease. Well used, this instinct becomes an early warning signal guarding against illness.

It turns out that the traditional yogic beliefs about balance between the two sides of our bodies contain some basic scientific truth. Inner tension and emotional stress can unbalance us physically, just as physical injuries can. Communication between the two sides of the body gets interrupted, our bodies go out of balance, and we show it in our postures and movements. When this happens we no longer walk with grace in our steps. Breathwalk has the power to repattern the muscles in our bodies, rebalancing their strength.

Scientific testing leads to similar conclusions. In the science of applied kinesiology, doctors use muscle testing to search for muscle imbalance between the two sides of the body. Any detected imbalance points toward potential problems with posture or even the health of various internal body organs. Kinesiologists have developed four postural measures for general good health that we can feel and see.

The Four Postural Measures for General Good Health
• Flexibility and a good range of bodily motion exist.

- The muscles on opposite sides of the body are of near equal strength.
- Opposite pairs of muscles balance the gait when walking.
- The muscles on the skull and in the lower spine that facilitate the motions of breathing are synchronized.

When we meet these four postural measures, our bodies have proper balance. We have an aesthetically pleasing flow as we walk and radiate beauty and strength. Our first impression to others is wellness, attractiveness, and comfort.

Over the years we have discovered that as we help people align and correct their walking style with the body scan, their posture and appearance also change. Their first impressions begin to reflect a basic inner vitality and health. According to Dr. Goodheart's quote, this must mean that Breathwalk works to repattern our muscles and to rebalance their strength. We decided to formally test out these observations and got some clear results.

When we ran some tests on thirty-five Breathwalkers using the precise measuring instruments of the kinesiologists, we found that our participants improved their performances remarkably on the first two measures after doing only one Breathwalk experience. Flexibility increased 20–50 percent. Muscle conditions went from twenty-eight imbalanced muscles to only one after a fifteen-minute Blissful Eagle Breathwalk. Strolling alone had eliminated some muscle imbalance (from twenty-eight to twenty), but Breathwalk reduced the incidences of muscle imbalance to almost zero.

In another set of tests, we tracked the balance of muscles that affect a good walking gait in our participants, the third postural measure of general good health. We initially found that 22 percent of the participants had some gait mechanism impairment, although none had serious impairments. These imbalances are the kind of impairment that all of us accumulate from stress, and we found that a single Lion Breathwalk of twenty minutes corrected all of these problems.

There are a number of things that can cause the skull-to-sacrum motion—the fourth measure—to get out of tune. Trauma to the head, whiplash, prolonged tension, jaw or bite problems, and drugs are some of them. Marijuana use in particular often causes a long-term disruption of movements at the base of the skull, which in turn contributes to memory problems and erratic motivation levels. Correcting the skull-sacrum movement helps people recover from the ill effects of such drugs. We have found that Breathwalk corrects this problem as it gradually restores full movement in most instances. Perhaps freeing motion in this crucial area also adds some of the "glow" that people show at the end of a good Breathwalk.

Brain Activity

Yogic tradition teaches that different patterns of breath used together with primal sounds triggers different modules of the brain. The ancients, the healers, and the yogis thought of the brain as having many different functional parts and networks—the two hemispheres plus many segments within each hemisphere. Different mental capacities would use different combinations of those parts. The yogis actually examined and classified how we do this and how we can enhance our brain functions with exercise, breathing, and attention. Now in the West, we have started using brain scanning and imagery to help us understand and directly observe how we use our brain in common tasks and during illness.

Does something great really happen to your brain when you Breathwalk? We thought that it must, judging from the obvious results, and to find out, we did some testing a number of years ago through a group at the University of Arizona Medical Center. A volunteer agreed to have a brain scan done to show levels of activity in the brain's different areas during a normal walk and then during a Breathwalk. We used an imaging technique called a "PET scan." For this test the subject is injected with a radioactive isotope. The isotope collects and concentrates along with the concentrations of blood. The PET scan can then give a map of the brain's areas that have become activated during an activity.

We had the volunteer walk normally for forty-five minutes. Then the researchers did a PET scan to see how the brain functioned. At the same time the next day, the volunteer did a Breathwalk for forty-five minutes. Again we had a PET scan done. The Breathwalk scans showed a 70–80 percent increase in the use of the parietal and temporal areas on the right side of the brain, increases in areas related to executive attention functions, and in areas on both sides in the prefrontal cortex. The scans also showed increased metacognition—more activity in the area of the insula and more integration of the two hemispheres based on the number of areas involved in both sides.

The experiment was only a first look. But it showed that a small change in the pattern of breathing changed areas of the brain related to cognitive function, judgment, and feelings, in addition to the areas related to movement and large muscles. Looking at the areas that were most activated tells us that after a Breathwalk we can focus our attention more effectively—even for multiple thoughts. We are clearer about our internal processes. And we can process thoughts and emotions with a more refined sense of their context.

Our research and that of others has revealed some of the changes that the yogis sensed. We'll need more tests to map out the differences between the various modes of brain activity induced by the different Breathwalk patterns, and to that end we have recently begun to work with researchers at the Mind/Body Medical Institute and Dr. Herbert Benson on a series of basic tests using fMRI. The fMRI is a type of magnetic scanning device that shows the fluctuations of oxygen used by tissue in the brain and elsewhere. Using this we can see how specific brain areas change activity as we use different breathing patterns and enter different states of meditation. We hope to find clues as to why the small changes in patterns of breathing and use of primal sounds lead to such different states of awareness and why Breathwalkers experience such strong mental clarity. Preliminary results are very encouraging and show a wide and complex array of changes. You don't have to master all of the science behind this, however, to tap into the benefits of Breathwalk. Just do it. The experience and benefits will remain all yours, even as the wheels of science turn slowly to discover the mechanisms of how Breathwalk works piece by piece and step by step.

Mood Changes

Psychologists have recently rediscovered the importance of moods to the quality of our daily lives. For decades the focus had remained upon behaviors and perceptions. Mood and emotions were considered peripheral and too intangible to base a science on. But since the early 1980s moods and emotions have regained a more central position. We have begun to understand how moods impact our feelings, thinking, memory, and health.

Here are some of the findings about the impact of moods on our lives. Some of them may surprise you; some you have known all along. Later we will show you the results of our surveys on how Breathwalk impacts our moods.

We remember feelings and ideas similar to the mood we are in. We remember things best when we are in the same mood that we were in when we learned them. This shows up in test anxiety. When you learn things in a calm state and then are tested when you are in an anxious state, you have difficulty remembering what you know. We notice more negative things when depressed and more positive things when elated. Similarly, our feelings of self-worth change with our mood states.

Positive moods enhance creativity. How you perceive yourself changes with mood. Good moods lead to positive expectations and optimism about the future. Bad moods equally lead to fear of failure, lack of confidence, and actions based upon the immediate future. Elevated moods and higher awareness produce a greater sense of control and choice over impulses related to food, drugs, and sex. Learning and skill improvement work best in positive mood states, with moderate to high arousal levels. Satisfaction in human relationships depends crucially upon each partner's ability to match the moods of the other. Creating rapport based in positive mood states enhances relationships; the accurate reading of the other person's mood, positive or negative, strengthens relationships.

Now, using brain imagery technology, we can document connections between the mood we are in and the brain areas that support that mood. However, the most important link we can form is between our awareness, our breath, and our moods. The breath can command the brain, and the brain can regulate our moods. This gives us a way to practically direct moods. That is how Breathwalk talks directly to our moods.

The "Common Colds" of Mood—
Anxiety and Depression

Anxiety and depression have become the "common colds" of moods. They are what psychologists and psychiatrists are most often called to treat. Research in the last few years has shown an alarming increase in both of these moods and a disturbing increase of their impact on the emotional and economic foundations of our lives.

Anxiety is the most common mood problem. It is characterized by excessive thinking, worry, and doubt that turns daily life into a flurry of fears and cautions. Thoughts dwell on the negative possibilities of what might happen and get caught into vicious circles of increasing concern. Once caught in this cycle, its victims often become depressed about the hopelessness of things. It affects about 4 percent of the population (8 percent if we include social anxiety)—over twenty-three million people in the United States are affected by these debilitating illnesses each year. Anxiety disorders cost the United States $46.6 billion in 1990 in direct and indirect costs, nearly one-third of the nation's total mental health bill of $148 billion. This figure continues to rise significantly each year.

Depression is characterized by a general feeling of lethargy, passivity, hopelessness, despair, low self-esteem, and alienation. The National Institute of Mental Health estimates that depression affects as many as twenty million Americans at any one time. Twenty-five percent of Americans will suffer from depression at least once during their lifetime. And twenty-five percent of the population suffers from mild winter seasonal affective disorder, with 5 percent suffering severely.

Several broad surveys conclude that depression in America has increased ten- to twentyfold in this century! If you were born after World War II, you are ten times more likely to be depressed than people born fifty years earlier. People born after 1950 are twenty times more likely to be depressed than those born before 1910. A cross-generation survey has found depression rates increasing in each generation. The World Health Organization's recent global assessment of the practical impact of every physical and mental factor on the quality of life has found that the "most surprising but solid trend is a massive increase in debilitating depression—non-polar, major incident depression. It is leaping to number two on the list of burdensome disease problems. In terms of estimated lost years of healthy life (measured by a new statistic called DALY, "disability adjusted life years"), it moves from 50.8 million to 78.7 million by 2020."* That means 78.7 million life years will be lost due to depression.

What has brought on this epidemic rise in anxiety and depression? Students of the modern wave of depression suggest that a complex blend of factors are to blame,

---

* This number refers to the millions of life years that are lost to depression.

including poor strategies for controlling our own moods, decreased exercise, increased passive viewing of television, increased drug usage (from alcohol to LSD), information overload, and high-fat, high-calorie diets. We personally believe that the loss of contact with our spiritual nature has much to do with it as well.

What can be done to forestall such damaging moods? Regular exercise, such as Breathwalking, can effectively change your mood and reconnect you to your sources of motivation. Dr. Robert E. Thayer in his 1997 book, *The Origin of Everyday Moods: Managing Energy, Tension, and Stress,* reports a simple and direct study where he compared the moods of people before and after either a fifteen-minute walk or after eating an apple. The walk proved more effective. In a study of addicted smokers and snackers, a short walk improved moods and reduced cravings by over 50 percent. Furthermore, the studies show that inducing a change of mood through walking keeps the changed mood in place much longer than through food, hypnosis, or other manipulations.

Our experience has shown that you can conquer the most common forms of anxiety and moderate depression with an appropriate program of Breathwalk. Producing change this way makes you stronger, more self-reliant, and more resilient. If you already live in generally positive mood states, we are convinced that Breathwalk can make life even better.

Measuring Breathwalk's Impact on Mood

We wanted to measure just how effective Breathwalk really is for tuning up moods to check our subjective observations. So we did some testing to find out. First we created some testing tools—specifically a mood chart and a mood map. The mood chart allowed our volunteers to report their own strength of feeling on thirty mood-related emotions. The mood map summarized the mood chart's information into negative, positive, and masterful mood components.

We tested two groups of people—participants from Cambridge, Massachusetts, and seminar attendees at the Anthony Robbins Life Mastery University in Maui. The Cambridge group comes closer to representing a sample of average adult Americans; the Robbins group all fell into the category of high achievers. We wanted to see what effects Breathwalk would have upon mood for both average and high achieving groups. In order to do this, we did mood maps for each group both before and after they did a Breathwalk.

Before Breathwalk, the Cambridge group was ruled by moderate negative feelings, as the "Before" left-hand column of the map shows. Negative moods somewhat outweighed positive ("Before" middle column) and masterful ("Before" right column) feelings. Group members also showed low arousal states—difficulty in engaging with life—and feelings of heaviness and irritation. After doing a single Breathwalk, the Cambridge participants again reported their strength of feeling about their moods. Look at the changes shown in the three "After" columns. A

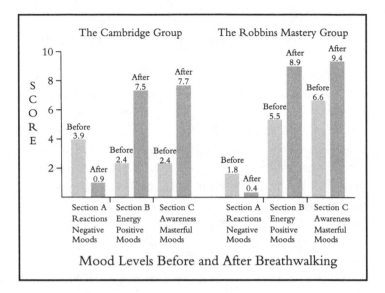

Mood Levels Before and After Breathwalking

single Breathwalk reduced negative moods by 80 percent and increased both positive and masterful moods by 70 percent. Negative and depressive trends in mood disappeared, and group members showed arousal and energy level increases.

People in the Anthony Robbins Life Mastery University reported a very different pattern of "before" and "after" results, with the same overall trend toward improved mood state. Remember that these people were generally either very high achievers in life already or they were strongly motivated by Tony's seminar. We wanted to see if Breathwalk could boost their already positive mood states.

The Robbins group started with a dominant positive and masterful mood. They were very open to life and full of energy and showed only small amounts of anxiety and scatteredness in their mental focus. Doing Breathwalk reduced their already low level of negative feelings to the negligible point. They also increased their sense of elevated positive feelings by 40 percent and masterful feelings by 30 percent.

What should we conclude from this research? Breathwalk works very effectively to diminish negative mood states and boost positive ones and develop moods for mastery. The physiological shifts we can create with Breathwalk gradually build an easily accessible and stable base for positive moods. With that base we can feel, examine, and learn from all our feelings—happiness and sadness, generosity and greediness, jealousy and contentment. The end result?

The Common Thread

You may wonder if there is any common thread that ties all of these effects together. The common thread for many of the effects we have documented is the fact that Breathwalk can adjust the main functions of the autonomic nervous system. This means that it can modify long-held tension and adjust the rhythms and function of the breath, heart rate, circulation, and other core processes in the body. Breathwalk embodies the code for exactly how to use breath and sound to create these specific changes. Many of the best benefits begin with the release of tension.

The yogic tradition teaches us that tension held in the body can become the root source of many of our health and fitness problems. When we hold tension within the body, we burn up large amounts of energy just staying tense—we're spinning our wheels and going nowhere. The yogis knew this many years ago, although they did not understand human physiology in the same way that we do today. Without the scientific terms we rely on today, they used their refined perception. Their observations have become compass points for directions to apply amazing new instruments and extensive analysis in a scientific manner.

Tension is stored in muscles. You can prove that for yourself. Think back to a time when you carried so much tension that some of your muscles literally ached. Science found quite a while ago that we possess two sorts of muscle tissue—striated and nonstriated. The striated muscles, such as our biceps, move our body members. They can exert tremendous force but tire quickly. They have to relax and rest. The nonstriated sort, the smooth muscles such as those in our arteries, are designed to hold on for long, long periods of time—literally to hold on for life. Those muscles have a learning capacity. Once they have learned to tense up in a certain way, they'll stay that way until some unlearning happens. It's like the twists in a length of rope. Once the rope strands learn how to be twisted and hold the tension, they stay that way.

Because of this ability, nonstriated muscles can become tension storage areas. When our emotionally driven tensions get expressed in these muscles, they learn it and just hold it, maybe for years and years. Our behavior can become seemingly programmed and rigid, robotic in nature. And that's not what these muscles are designed for. All this holding of emotional tensions not only wastes our store of energy, it hurts us. Somehow we need to learn how to release the tension stored up in our bodies' muscles.

Where does all this tension originate? In fear. And while it may be helpful to seek out the sources of our fears through counseling, one of the wonderful aspects of Breathwalk is that it has the capability to rather quickly remove the effects of fear from our bodies. When we release the tension within us, we have more energy to use productively.

Perhaps science will trace out the pathways by which we can affect the autonomic system and the brain and find mechanisms for the release of toxic tension. In the end it will map the mechanisms that let us become relaxed, centered, and happy—to be a human being as we fulfill our destiny one step at a time.

Points to Remember

- When Breathwalk creates a signature of wellness in the body, it can be detected physically in the following: heart and body rhythms that show increased complexity and a "fractal-like" pattern in their variation, the ability of the eyes to focus narrowly or widely with speed and clarity, the measurable balance of the muscles, and enhanced brain functions.
- The release of inner tension held in the smooth muscles of the body may well be the common thread that links many of these vitality effects in Breathwalk.
- Although the frequency of disruptive moods and mood disorders is rising rapidly, we can easily manage our moods with regular exercise and particularly Breathwalk.

Conclusion

A GREAT COACH MOTIVATED HIS TEAM WITH the phrase "Exercise with attitude!" We say to our Breathwalkers, "Exercise with attitude and altitude." The attitude is to relax, enjoy, and be fully present. The altitude is being aware and seeing yourself for the beauty, spirit, and potential that you possess. If you doubt yourself or forget all the resources you have in your design, you fight your own vitality.

There are three things we like to remember that give the perfect attitude and altitude for a Breathwalk. First, we always have a choice. That is one of our great gifts as human beings. We can change our own state. We can be sad or happy. We can create a good habit or a bad one. We can increase or decrease our awareness. We can think only of this moment or stretch our mind through centuries. We can even create habits that make us aware and give us more choice over our habits.

Second, we have everything we need to make those choices. We lack nothing, and we are not broken. We can call on resources within and without to reach our goals. We have everything we need for a rich and happy life inside us. We are receptacles of millions of years of evolution, filled up with skills and talents and dormant powers. We are part of the universe, and just like the rest of the universe, we begin with energy and light. Then we evolve as rhythm, movement, and finally awareness.

The structure of our mind and body is crafted with infinite subtlety by the touch of the Divine to let us use all these resources. Sometimes we forget this.

We are often told the answers to our problems are outside. Take a pill, buy this or that, or search for some miracle worker. It's certainly true that we have better pills, more things to buy, and more skilled professionals than in times past. But we all have the ability to call on our own healing energy, insight, commitment, and action to create happiness and perpetual success. Each time we find a way to connect to our inner resources and use them to express our heart and excel at life, we increase our vitality. We open the door to our spirit, and we shield ourselves from many physical and emotional ailments.

Third, we are spiritual beings here to have a human experience. We are neither animals nor angels. We bring the heavens to the earth through our actions, and we transform the earth to the heavens with our prayer and compassion.

Breathwalk

We live in this intricate mesh of heaven and earth woven through our senses and awareness. When our body and mind are balanced, we can easily feel who we are and know what we want to do.

We are designed so that body and mind each affect the other in precise and powerful patterns. If you move your body in certain ways, you move your feelings. If you breathe a certain way, you fill your self with a sense of the spirit. If you hold certain thoughts, you cloud or clear the mind to sense the world. The beauty of this intricate mesh of body, mind, and spirit is that we can nourish our whole selves through breath.

Our Body of Light

All through this book we are aware of the spiritual dimension of Breathwalk and other forms of meditative walking. Many people have asked us why they feel so expanded and at peace after a good Breathwalk. Some people report feeling a great energy or light around them. A few also report that they can literally see a glow. There is a basis to these experiences, well-known to every spiritual tradition and school of wisdom. We want to touch on it here so you have an introduction to how Breathwalk impacts your spirit.

When people are filled with spirit, a wonderful thing occurs—radiance. The characteristics and mechanisms of that subtle radiance give us a link between body, mind, and spirit. Saintly people and healers commonly project an aura that we can visibly see. This is the light body. Each of us can sense or intuit our own light body like a surrounding glow that is part of our presence. It varies its shape, color, and motion with changes in our health, mental state, and spiritual status. Walking, especially Breathwalking, works as one powerful way to induce changes in the light body. This in turn opens our mental and emotional sensitivity to the spirit.

The light body has a diameter, which some people can visibly see. It extends all around the physical body in an oval-like shape. It swirls with many colors. If we just look at how far it radiates, we can tell a lot. Radiance that projects between 1 1/2 to 3 feet out from the physical body evenly on all sides shows balance, but with little sensitivity. With such a light body we become vulnerable to even small emotional bursts from other people. It will be hard to maintain a sense of purpose and direction. As we get stronger the aura extends farther. It can extend as far as 9 feet in all directions, although that is unusual. At that size even the average onlooker can see or at least feel the aura.

The light body can be symmetrical or uneven and rough. Areas that radiate far less than others look like little depressions or dimples. Those dimples indicate our physical and emotional weak spots. The emotions associated with those areas, if not dealt with, can contribute to illness and to poor decision making.

The use of the breathing ratios in Breathwalk and the impact of the awakeners expand the aura and remove any blemish or weak spots. We can literally radiate more light. The extra radiance contributes to the feeling of presence and attraction others sense about us. It shields us from reacting to unwanted thoughts and emotions. It shines out as a light beacon that says more about our spirit and its condition than hundreds of books. In the inner eye of another person, in the sensitive subconscious, we become all brightness and light.

The flow of energy through the light body takes many

paths. One major path resembles a grand stream that flows from the crown of the head and down through seven pools along the centerline of the body. The yogis called these pools "chakras." The word means circle. The pools swirl in circles like whirlpools. They dance to ratios of the breath, to the projection of our awareness, and to ratios of clockwise and counterclockwise motions that inform the activity of our glands and nerves.

The chakras are lined up on the vertical axis of the body, near the base of the spine, the sex organ, the navel area, the heart, the throat, the brow point, the crown of the head, and all around the body like a shell. When we reach a fine, harmonious rhythm within us, these centers adjust their movements to the demand on them. Each activity we carry out activates a particular combination of chakras and areas of the body so we can perform well.

Caroline Myss, in her widely sold 1996 book, *Anatomy of the Spirit: The Seven Stages of Power and Healing,* links the condition of chakras and the light body to numerous ailments and shows how emotional agendas relate to them. By her own direct observations, "Your physical body is surrounded by an energy field. . . . It is both an information center and a highly sensitive perceptual system. We are constantly in communication with everything around us through this system. . . . Each organ and system in the body is calibrated to absorb and process specific emotional and psychological energies. That is, each area of the body transmits energy on a specific detailed frequency, and when we are healthy, all are in tune. An area of the body that is not transmitting at its normal frequency indicates the location of the problem." The chakras and the condition of the light body reveal what is happening within us—how healthy we are, how much in conflict we feel, and how much we dwell with our spirit.

What happens when we use Breathwalk to strengthen the spirit and increase the brightness of our light bodies? Breathwalk opens the flows within the chakras. It prepares body and mind to host the spirit. It heightens awareness by removing energy blocks. The use of the primal sound scales unlocks fixations in the chakras as the breathing ratios expand the aura and open the meridians. The permutations and combinations of the primal sounds unlock the potentials in the light body and the psyche.

It works in a gradual, steady process. Each step generates and releases a little more energy. With each step the chakras move more freely and shine a bit more. With each step your soul gains a clearer voice to guide you toward your true destination.

Walking with the Strength of the Spirit

We are not the first to walk for health, well-being, and inspiration. We join a line of people millions long that stretches to the beginning of our records and beyond. You might draw some inspiration from the amazing efforts of other people who have walked, opened their hearts, and lived to their full spirit and potential over the centuries.

Walking and spirit go together. Walking of any kind has always been a spiritual, soulful activity. It clears the mind, sorts out emotional turmoil, lifts our mood, and can reconnect us to the vastness of nature.

A walk puts us in touch with the human scale of time. It adds a moment of perspective to our thinking. It creates a space where we can gather our body and mind until we are fully present and aware. It is then that we can engage the uplifting powers of the spirit and wrestle with the urgent and sometimes dark messages we get about the need to change ourselves.

For thousands of years spiritual guides and saints of the world have used walking in astounding ways. Those spiritual masters and aspirants paved the way for all of us to invite spirit into our lives. The practices of those masters of the spirit can inspire us now. We need not repeat the daunting feats of discipline and rigor they performed. We can capture most of the effects and the best qualities of what they did using the Breathwalk. Breathwalk can be used to develop courage, discipline, healing ability, and spiritual states.

Fire Walking

It is true that in many cultures some people—usually priests, healers, or warriors—developed the practice of walking over fire. They would prepare themselves, change their inner state through prayer, purification, or group practices, and then walk unharmed across ten to thirty feet of glowing hot coals. The purpose of such things had nothing to do with the fire or the hot coals. It was all about fear. It was about beliefs. It was about our ability to walk past the barriers in life we create with fear within our own minds.

Just imagine what your mind would bring up when you actually stand before a bed of hot coals. You smell the burning wood. You feel the hot wind hit your legs and face. You see the crackling coals turning a falling leaf to cinder.

Now you will walk on this? Doubts, fears, and reevaluations of how you got here are natural.

Suppose you reach deep within and summon forth calmness, joy, and steadiness. You are ready to embrace whatever experience happens. If you can do it here, you can do it other places. You go beyond fear and get new choices. The capacity to make decisions without reactive fear constitutes the stuff of leadership and extraordinary living. When you stand before other things that may burn and consume you, you can act with the feelings you need to go ahead. Walking past our fears touches the spirit by casting aside limitations and creating openness.

The Running Buddhists of Mt. Hiei

Starting in the late 800s, followers of Tendai Buddhism in Japan developed a practice that is both grueling and fascinating: To purify themselves, the monks did a run-walk marathon. The routes varied from eighteen to fifty-two miles without rest and with little food. They learned to stop for only a few seconds, perhaps a minute at a time, at over 255 stations of worship to perform specific meditations and prayers for ancestors, for purification, and for the benefit of all people. On a typical marathon the disciple recited those prayers, negotiated thousands of stairs, climbed steep mountain slopes, suffered through all kinds of weather in traditional sparse garments, and walked with a meditative attitude on each step.

Honor came from performing this marathon. The follower had to qualify physically, mentally, and spiritually. The task itself became a transformative experience in which all attachments were left behind and the follower simply stood in service before reality.

When the monks reached readiness, they engaged in a full one hundred days of the same daily marathon. They reported that the hardest task was not eating little or strengthening the muscles, but learning to keep the right posture, head up and balanced and looking slightly ahead. They had to maintain constant attention, alertness, and balance over every terrain and in all kinds of weather. If they qualified, they entered a severe training over a period of seven years. During that training they ran a marathon for a thousand days.

To succeed, they had to learn secrets of the breath and rhythm—as you will learn the secrets of Breathwalk in more moderate, enjoyable exercises.

What did these aspirants gain? All reports said they gained incredible clarity, sensitivity, and radiance. Their eyes shone so brightly, they were said to heal just by looking at someone. They became compassionate, humble, and active in the joy of life. They sought an ordeal of transformation to affirm their capacity to live in the spirit now, to put aside petty fears and attachments, and to complete a sense of trust in their own spirit. The severity of the task is not what creates the transformation. It is the intensity of the awareness needed to do the task that powers such deep transfiguration.

The Wind Walkers of Tibet

In ancient Tibet, when that area still served as the university of spirit at the top of the world, people needed to communicate over very long distances and rugged territory.

Many early explorers to these regions witnessed and recorded the famous *lung-gom-pa* walkers. They would fly over the ground as if on the wind. They would cover two hundred miles or more and travel without rest for two or three days. They would travel faster than horses and yet seem to glide over the ground as if weightless. To train in this tradition, aspiring wind walkers had to first qualify by being able to sit, to visualize, to control the breath, and to develop concentration.

Then the aspirants would receive training in *traatik,* a form of gazing meditation where they fixed their eyes upon an object such as the tip of the nose, a geometric figure, or a star. They would leave all other distractions and then create a rhythm of movement of the breath. The wind walkers also used certain well-guarded mantras. All this was employed in their walking practices.

Their real goal still remained the same as that of other monks, to walk lightly upon the earth and carry all burdens with joy and victory. They attained this by cultivating the secrets of the breath and the neutral mind from meditations just as in the inner walks that we will teach you.

Guru Nanak's Sacred Journeys

Guru Nanak founded the Sikh way of life that we the authors follow. He taught and exemplified humility, service, and meditation upon God and the Naam, the sacred names of God. He went on several long journeys, walking all around India, up into China, down to Burma, and all the way over to Mecca. He walked, and with his faithful minstrel, Mardana, he imparted teachings through poetry, song, meditation, and healing. Every tradition acknowledged his radiance and presence.

As he covered these thousands of miles, he would walk and meditate upon the Naam and upon primal sounds with each step. He called the practice charan jappa—deep meditative repetition of a mantra with the feet. Anyone could join him. As he healed and inspired, he asked people to elevate themselves—to see the spirit in every person, not just in a special class or religion. He mastered the inner currents of sound and the power of the breath's rhythm. Each of his words became potent to heal.

One of his favored walks was what we here call the Dove Breathwalk, which has an 8/8 rhythm: eight steps as you inhale and eight steps as you exhale. He used the sound SAT KARTAR as he walked. It means "The true One That Is is the true Doer of all." He repeated SAT with one step and KARTAR with the next. That walk makes a person relaxed, open, humble, and constantly aware of dwelling in the hand of God.

Nine Sikh teachers or gurus followed after Guru Nanak. The last, Guru Gobind Singh, shone as a poet, linguist, warrior, healer, and leader extraordinaire. He had to train soldiers that could defend his followers and other defenseless groups from Moghul persecution. Using yoga, physical training, and tools like Breathwalk, he transformed common people into a force with amazing endurance.

They walked tirelessly for miles alongside the horses. They engaged in sword battles for twelve hours at a time without tiring, and they used swords that weighed as much as eighteen pounds. No one walked less than five miles a day to train for physical endurance, and all learned to call on their spirit for invincible vitality.

Spirit Walkers Everywhere

The drive to express our spirit and soul has seeded a spiritual walking heritage in every culture. Native Americans have a wonderful practice known as a vision walk—a quest to connect to the guides of the inner spirit realm. It involves one to many days of purification and meditation, often with solitude. Walking in natural sacred areas becomes part of the transformation. Many shamanic traditions use walking in meditation as part of training. When in the right state of mind and mood, a person can perceive the cues in the environment needed to learn healing. Pilgrims travel hundreds of miles along paths once traveled by a saint. For example, millions of pilgrims have trekked the five hundred miles from the French border and across northern Spain to reach the tomb of St. James. That pilgrimage route is called the Camino de Santiago.

For centuries such techniques remained closely guarded secrets. They were too revolutionary to teach widely in the rigid political environments. Elite yogis, healers, and spiritual seekers in diverse disciplines knew them. The knowledge was not available to the average person. In the past, those who wanted to learn about spirit had to make incredible sacrifices and enormous efforts.

Now we are crossing the threshold into a more global age, when awareness and spirit will be essential. This new time buzzes with rapid change, instant communication, diverse beliefs, and challenges. To thrive in it, we need ways to find our spiritual center in many little ways. In a short walk. In the normal course of work, home, and play. So Breathwalk and many other powerful techniques have now become widely available. These techniques are our heritage. They are essential tools to excel in and enjoy this next age of humanity.

Today we see many people in walkathons for hunger, for AIDS, for peace, for cancer, and for every other cause we can think of. Individuals have walked hundreds of thousands of miles, coast to coast, even, to raise money and awareness for their cause. We walk to inspire ourselves and others. We do it all the time—not just in faraway lands or distant times. Even if you have never tried it, start now to elevate others as well as yourself. Share a walk and share the breath of life.

Begin gradually. Breathwalk by yourself, with a partner, or in a group. It is time to learn what only experience itself can teach you. It is time to feel the motivation and energy that comes to your cells through every fiber of your body. Experience will uplift you and sustain you. It is that experience that makes you feel great.

As you practice the language of energy encoded in Breathwalk, you become radiant with vitality. Radiance that others feel as attraction. Radiance that the universe feels as presence. Radiance that invites in your spirit, its lessons, and its vitality to guide you on your path to fulfillment, enjoyment, and health.

Points to Remember

- Three attitudes: We always have a choice; we have everything we need to make those choices; and we are spiritual beings here to have an experience as a human being.
- The spirit within us all is as real as the body and as energetic as electricity, if we will only allow it to flow. The aura or light body that we project is a visible sign of the health of the spirit.
- The chakras are centers of energy in the body connected through the meridians. When the seven chakras are free to flow and adjust, not only does the light body grow, our energy and mental vitality increase as well.
- Breathwalk opens the flow of energy through the chakras, removes blockages, and unlocks the hidden potential in our bodies and our psyches.
- Walking has been used to naturally connect to our spirit for as long as we have records. Those who have come before us have performed great feats and left behind inspiring stories.

Breathwalk Programs Guide

EACH BREATHWALK PROGRAM IS OUTLINED so you can easily follow the five steps. You will find the detailed description of the awakeners and Breathwalk patterns referred to in the corresponding sections of this guide. For a complete description of the Innerwalks, refer back to chapter 9. Enjoy!

Health Care Alert

Our instructions and recommendations in the Breathwalk programs do not replace, but are intended to complement, regular physical and psychological expert health services.

Neglect of any serious symptom or not following through with regular checkups can be harmful to your health.

Before you start any program of exercise be sure to check with your physician and any other health care provider you work with. If you get any negative symptoms at all from breathing or exercise, check with your doctor. Do not push ahead blindly or ignore symptoms without advice. Our instructional programs do not replace diagnosis and careful monitoring by a professional who knows you individually.

Programs

Quick Start Energy Booster

If you ever had a day when meetings piled high and fatigue or distraction accompanied the pileup, then this is your magic wand. You have a short time and need to be able to sprint to the goal. Do this when you need to shake your body and mind out of a low-energy slumber. You want to be ready to act, focus, and take on a challenge. The exercises in the awakener give you immediate potency and activate an instinct to excel. Strong nerves and a good sexual energy are other benefits. The Hawk Breathwalk in this program builds your readiness for action, mental or physical, with increased confidence, optimism, and motivation. Many people in business or the performance arts use this Breathwalk to prepare for a presentation.

1. Awakener 3: Potency and Zeal
2. Align as you pace up to speed and scan your body.

3. Breathwalk 3: The Hawk (8/4 segmented breath)

Vitality Intervals

1st Interval	Hawk	3 minutes
	Normal Breathing	2 minutes
2nd Interval	Hawk	5 minutes
	Normal Breathing	2 minutes
3rd Interval	Hawk	7 minutes
	Normal Breathing	2 minutes

4. Balance as you pace down and shift your focus for 2 minutes. Then do the triple balance stretch.
5. Innerwalk: Sensory Bubble

Program 2

Rejuvenate Your Energy Reserves

Many times we need to apply our attention and energy to a task steadily for a long time, until it is done. If our basic reserves of energy are sufficient, we can stay the course and keep a sense of clarity and purpose about what we do. Many parents say they feel as though they dash here and there, cover one fire after another, but lose track of what they intended to do and become irritable. This program builds energy reserves and makes your mind steady. It takes pressure off your back and makes your spine more flexible.

As you increase your number and length of vitality intervals, feelings of irritation, pessimism, and scatteredness move toward calmness, openness, and clarity.

1. Awakener 1: Opening to Go
2. Align as you pace up to speed and scan your body.
3. Breathwalk 1: The Eagle (4/4 segmented breath)

Vitality Intervals

1st Interval	Eagle	3 minutes
	Normal Breathing	5 minutes
2nd and 3rd Intervals	Repeat 1st Interval	

4. a. Balance as you pace down and shift your focus for 2 minutes. Then do the triple balance stretch.
   b. Awakener 2: Hip and Spine Balance
5. Innerwalk: Sensory Bubble

Program 3

Gather Your Distributed Energy

Sometimes we have plenty of energy, but it is distributed in ways that make it unavailable. We lock it into tension, one part of us fighting another. We are prepared to move one way and the opposite way at the same time. Emotionally we are equally ready to trust someone and run away. Imagine walking and releasing each of those energy pools like hundreds of rivulets that all flow together in a great and steady wave to support you. This program releases stuck energies in your body and emotions. It replaces sadness with an inner strength and a feeling of confident contentment. You can sense new circulation to areas that were contracted and increase intensity and vigor. Unlike the first program, which builds your energy quickly and narrowly, this builds your energy like a rising tide until you are ready to apply it with easy steadiness.

1. Awakener 11: Letting Go
2. Align as you pace up to speed and scan your body.
3. Breathwalk 6: The Cheetah (8/4 complete deep breath)

Vitality Intervals

1st Interval	Cheetah	5 minutes
	Normal Breathing	3 minutes
2nd Interval	Cheetah	10 minutes
	Normal Breathing	3 minutes

4. Balance as you pace down and shift your focus for 2 minutes. Then do the triple balance stretch.
5. Innerwalk: Sensory Bubble

Simple Anxiety to Inner Calm

Anxiety is familiar. It comes in little ways, scratching at the edge of our awareness like kittens' claws. Occasionally it builds to a huge wave and commands our attention like a lion's roar—a full-fledged panic attack. Most of us fall between these two extremes and have moments of anxiety that do not paralyze us. They are like inner noise. They take away from our clear focus.

It is just like trying to give a speech when a critical friend comes in the back to watch. We can become so nervous about being watched that we lose track of our words. Or think how many people can shoot a basketball through the hoop easily on their own, then miss it as people stand around to watch. This is social anxiety. It is common in over 85 percent of us.

We can find the inner calm at the center of the anxiety. Then, even if we feel some nervousness, it doesn't bother us, and we can find that flow and natural expressiveness that comes when we are in charge and doing well.

1. Awakener 4: Relax and Center
2. Align as you pace up to speed and scan your body.
3. Breathwalk 1: The Eagle (4/4 segmented breath)

Vitality Intervals

1st Interval	Eagle	3 minutes
	Normal Breathing	5 minutes
2nd Interval	Eagle	5 minutes
	Normal Breathing	3 minutes
3rd Interval	Eagle	10 minutes
	Normal Breathing	1 minute

4. Balance as you pace down and shift your focus for 2 minutes. Then do the triple balance stretch.
5. Innerwalk: Sensory Bubble

Program 5

From Depression to Clear and Connected

Even if we are normally on an even keel, we can still suffer a transient depression. Depressions can come and go, and they can sometimes teach us important things about ourselves. However, when they stay too long and we do not understand why, our energy level plummets and we feel disconnected from the things that matter to us. Our relationships are often first to suffer. We feel isolated and alone no matter how many people we care for or who care about us.

We can lose motivation as our ability to imagine a

future collapses. Instead we are filled with inner talk that negates us, criticizes our efforts, or tells us how we are not worthy. We need a strong connection to our future, our dreams, and our destiny. The ability to switch out of this mood is essential. Staying depressed is harmful to our health and can block the expression of our spirit.

This Breathwalk program has helped thousands of people alleviate depression, learn what they need to know from it, and select feelings that give them the emotional resources they need.

1. Awakener 7: Better Moods
2. Align as you pace up to speed and scan your body.
3. Breathwalk 8: The Blissful Eagle (4/4 segmented/whispered breath)

Vitality Intervals

1st Interval	Blissful Eagle	5 minutes
	Normal Breathing	3 minutes
2nd Interval	Blissful Eagle	10 minutes
	Normal Breathing	3 minutes
3rd Interval	Blissful Eagle	5 minutes
	Normal Breathing	1 minute

4. a. Balance as you pace down and shift your focus for 2 minutes.
   b. Do breath of fire through the right nostril for 3 minutes.
5. Innerwalk: Walking the Breath for 2–3 minutes

Program 6

From Distracted, Busy, and Hyperactive
to Receptive and Intimate

Faxes, phone calls, e-mail, ads, letters, drop-ins, to-do lists, and everything else can make us feel as though we are walking through a swarm of pesky bugs. No matter how beautiful it is on our walk, it is hard to stay in a good mood and appreciate what we are doing.

Real pleasure comes when we can be relaxed and present rather than distracted. The best meeting is when we can become receptive and put aside the jumpy, put-out-the-fire mode we were in before the meeting. If we can switch this mood quickly and easily, we can communicate better, connect to other people, and form better teams.

1. Awakener 10: Being Present
2. Align as you pace up to speed and scan your body.
3. Breathwalks 1: The Eagle (4/4 segmented breath) and 2: The Dove (8/8 segmented breath)

Vitality Intervals

1st Interval	Eagle	5 minutes
	Normal Breathing	3 minutes
2nd Interval	Dove	5 minutes
	Normal Breathing	2 minutes
3rd Interval	Dove	10 minutes
	Normal Breathing	3 minutes

4. Balance as you pace down and shift your focus for 3 minutes. Then do the triple balance stretch.
5. Innerwalk: Play and Replay

*From Doubtful and Lethargic
to Motivated and Ready*

Life is so spectacular and changeable, it seems impossible to be weighted down with a feeling of lethargy and boredom or stopped from action by a surge of doubts. Still, it happens. When we succumb to doubt and hesitate as we wait for something "out there" to rescue or entertain us, we are, in fact, the source of the doubt, lethargy, and their attendant problems.

We need to get motivated, get focused, and take a leap forward. At such times we can call upon our inner resources and create change both inside and outside. We have a core of joy. We need to shake off any dullness and let it through. This program cuts to that core and gives you the power to move ahead with confidence.

1. Awakener 8: Pure Joy
2. Align as you pace up to speed and scan your body.
3. Breathwalk 3: The Hawk (8/4 segmented breath)

Vitality Intervals

1st Interval	Hawk	3 minutes
	Normal Breathing	2 minutes
2nd Interval	Hawk	5 minutes
	Normal Breathing	2 minutes
3rd Interval	Hawk	7 minutes
	Normal Breathing	1 minute

4. Balance as you pace down and shift your focus for 2 minutes. Then do the triple balance stretch.
5. Innerwalk: Gathering Your Senses

Program 8

Mental Clarity

Mental clarity in this program comes from a blend of alertness, profound calmness, and vivid awareness in the present. We open the lungs and stimulate the circulation. Then the Eagle Breathwalk adds alertness and a positive mood. We switch to a Tiger Breathwalk pattern for strength, calmness, and the ability to drop any anxiety or distractions.

Any time you need a sense of openness, wide peripheral vision, and enhanced sensitivity to see a situation lucidly, do this program.

1. Awakener 10: Being Present
2. Align as you pace up to speed and scan your body.
3. Breathwalks 1: The Eagle (4/4 segmented breath) and
   5: The Tiger (8/8 complete deep breath)

Vitality Intervals

1st Interval	Eagle	3 minutes
	Normal Breathing	2 minutes
2nd Interval	Eagle	5 minutes
	Normal Breathing	3 minutes
3rd Interval	Tiger	5 minutes
	Normal Breathing	3 minutes

4. Balance as you pace down and shift your focus for 2 minutes. Then do the triple balance stretch.
5. Innerwalk: Play and Replay

Intuition

We can all use a little intuition. Intuition lets us recognize things that we know but are outside of our normal awareness. It lets us apply our wisdom and years of experience in a new situation. We pick up on the little cues that signal danger and can keep us safe. Mostly we think of things in terms of stereotypes of broad categories instead of seeing them directly, as they are. The ability to see something on its own terms and use its uniqueness is also intuition.

1. Awakener 9: Intuitively Right
2. Align as you pace up to speed and scan your body.
3. Breathwalks 5: The Tiger (8/8 complete deep breath) and 8: The Blissful Eagle (4/4 segmented/whispered breath)

Vitality Intervals

1st Interval	Tiger	3 minutes
	Normal Breathing	2 minutes
2nd Interval	Tiger	5 minutes
	Normal Breathing	3 minutes
3rd Interval	Blissful Eagle	10 minutes
	Normal Breathing	3 minutes

4. Balance as you pace down and shift your focus for 2 minutes. Then do the triple balance stretch.
5. Innerwalk: Sensory Bubble

Program 10

Focus

A well-known therapist estimated that 40 percent of our normal neuroses and worry would go away if we learned how to focus. Our mind catches us in the grips of fear, sadness, and anxiety by fixating its focus too close to or too far from something. When we Breathwalk and we switch our focus from the vitality intervals to the balance step, we train our focus capacity and drop many mind-sets that keep us captive. We induce a new openness with a shift of focus.

How many times have you had a problem that seemed like a mountain? Then one more piece of information or an idea and suddenly it is just a little problem, a molehill, in a much larger landscape. This program gives the focus to you instead of to your problems or to your mind's fantasies.

1. Awakener 5: New Lungs
2. Align as you pace up to speed and scan your body.
3. Breathwalks 3: The Hawk (8/4 segmented breath) and 2: The Dove (8/8 segmented breath)

Vitality Intervals

1st Interval	Hawk	3 minutes
	Normal Breathing	2 minutes
2nd Interval	Repeat 1st Interval	
3rd Interval	Dove	5 minutes
	Normal Breathing	2 minutes
4th Interval	Hawk	5 minutes
	Normal Breathing	3 minutes

4. Balance as you pace down and shift your focus for 2 minutes. Then do the triple balance stretch.
5. Innerwalk: Play and Replay

Program 11

Learn and Create

The manager of a computer product division told us, "Everything I learned five years ago is either obsolete or changed completely by new things that have been added. To stay on top of my job, not even to get ahead, it's like I go to school every day and I still have homework to do when I go home."

In this age of learning, speed and continuous retraining is the rule. It is as true for the secretary as for the engineer, for the therapist as for the minister, and for the tradesman as for the politician. To move ahead, we need to be creative as well as to learn.

Fortunately we now know the brain keeps learning and can be creative through our life span as long as we stimulate it and keep using it. The exercises of Breathwalk are ideal for getting the brain in shape to take on this new age of information with a smile. The use of the primal sounds is especially effective at sorting out thoughts and keeping us away from overload.

1. Awakener 7: Better Moods
2. Align as you pace up to speed and scan your body.
3. Breathwalks 10: The Radiant Hawk (8/4 segmented/whispered breath) and
1: The Eagle (4/4 segmented breath)

Vitality Intervals

1st Interval	Radiant Hawk	3 minutes
	Normal Breathing	3 minutes
2nd Interval	Radiant Hawk	5 minutes
	Normal Breathing	2 minutes
3rd Interval	Eagle	5 minutes
	Normal Breathing	3 minutes

4. Balance as you pace down and shift your focus for 2 minutes. Then do the triple balance stretch.

5. Innerwalk: Sensory Bubble

Program 12

Rapport

Two young lovers were sitting on a park bench. A vendor passed by, selling ice cream and balloons. It was amazing to watch them select two kinds of ice cream and several balloons, including one shaped to look like a bird, without uttering a word. It was a nod here, a wink there, accented with a shrug, a touch, and a kiss. They were in rapport. People who watched only smiled and often gave a quick affirmative squeeze of the hand to their partners. Rapport means instant communication, a trust and emotional affinity that makes words too slow.

When we are in rapport the world seems close and cozy. We feel understood. We break that rapport with inner dissent, distrust, and anxiety. If we create it within ourselves, we can easily open and extend it to others. It is the primary glue in our feelings of connectedness and the healing that those feelings bring.

1. Awakener 11: Letting Go
2. Align as you pace up to speed and scan your body.
3. **a.** Breathwalk 8: The Blissful Eagle (4/4 segmented/whispered breath)

Vitality Intervals

1st Interval	Blissful Eagle	5 minutes
	Normal Breathing	5 minutes
2nd Interval	Blissful Eagle	5 minutes

b. Awakener 1: Opening to Go
c. Breathwalk 5: The Tiger (4/4 complete deep breath)

Vitality Intervals

1st Interval	Tiger	3 minutes
	Normal Breathing	5 minutes
2nd Interval	Tiger	5 minutes

4. Balance as you pace down and shift your focus for 2 minutes. Then do the triple balance stretch.
5. Innerwalk: Sensory Bubble (Note: When you do the bubble exercise at the end, you may wish to hold your partner's hands and start with your eyes wide open, looking at each other; then close your eyes and expand the senses.)

Consistency

This program is a simple way to feel an emotional and spiritual continuity between one moment and the next and between all your inner parts. It is normal to split ourselves into many functional parts. It is not normal for all of them to conflict and result in inconsistent and inconsiderate behaviors and impulses. This Breathwalk consolidates you more and more as you increase the times and numbers of the intervals. When we become consistent to ourselves, we can speak truth easily and create trust that holds relationships together.

1. Awakener 6: Spinal Flex
2. Align as you pace up to speed and scan your body.
3. a. Breathwalk 7: The Lion (4/4/4 complete deep breath)

Vitality Intervals

1st Interval	Lion	3 minutes
	Normal Breathing	3 minutes
2nd and 3rd Intervals	Repeat 1st Interval	

    b. Awakener 4: Relax and Center
4. Balance as you pace down and shift your focus for 2 minutes. Then do the triple balance stretch.
5. Innerwalk: Gathering Your Senses

Program 14

Integrity

Integrity calls on courage and on recognition of what is important to us. It calls on our character and sense of value. By acknowledging what is of true importance, we can treat everything that arises from within and without in the appropriate manner. We have an integrity that forges an identity.

If we recognize and act on our own identity, we can recognize the identity and values of others. We can begin to uncover some of the simple truths and secrets of nature as well.

This program can help you increase the awareness of your integrity and your capacity to hold to doing what is most important.

1. Awakener 8: Pure Joy
2. Align as you pace up to speed and scan your body.
3. Breathwalk 9: The Intuitive Dove (8/8 segmented/whispered breath)

Vitality Intervals

1st Interval	Intuitive Dove	3 minutes
	Normal Breathing	3 minutes
2nd Interval	Intuitive Dove	5 minutes
	Normal Breathing	3 minutes
3rd Interval	Intuitive Dove	5 minutes
	Normal Breathing	3 minutes

4. Balance as you pace down and shift your focus for 2 minutes. Then do the triple balance stretch.
5. Innerwalk: Walking the Breath

Program 15

Emotional Presence

This program opens your heart and helps you drop unnecessary defensiveness. It calms you and even helps to detoxify your body so you can relax and become present.

A woman was attending an annual gala party. She stood near a window, tapping one foot and moving her hands nervously on a railing. I asked: "Where are you?" Momentarily startled, she said, "I was all over. My mind was at last year's party, when my husband was alive. Then I was at the marathon I am going to run in a few weeks. And I was full of other thoughts." We both chuckled. She became present and then walked away from the window with us to enjoy the gala.

That is the secret. We stay emotionally absent by letting the past be in the present and running from the present into the future or into our fantasies. That is why it is so central a practice in many spiritual traditions to become present in the here and now.

When we are in the present we can express ourselves and connect with our life in a satisfying and rich manner. A big part of being present is simply letting go. This Breathwalk program helps your mind and body detoxify and eliminate ill thoughts and feelings so you can open to the present with emotional vigor.

Breathwalk

1. Awakener 12: Loving Feelings
2. Align as you pace up to speed and scan your body.
3. Breathwalk 4: The Owl (4/8 segmented breath)

Vitality Intervals

1st Interval	Owl	3 minutes
	Normal Breathing	3 minutes
2nd Interval	Owl	5 minutes
	Normal Breathing	3 minutes

4. Balance as you pace down and shift your focus for 2 minutes. Then do the triple balance stretch.
5. Inner Walk: Whole Brain Cinema

Program 16

Spiritual Abundance

One of the first sensations that comes with an elevated spirit is the feeling of abundance. When we are disconnected from our spirit it is easy to live in scarcity. Then our minds fill with fears and block our opportunities.

We were at lunch with a very socially accomplished and wealthy student. We had left our cash behind. She knew it. So she tried to prove that our abundance depended on her—that without her fortunes, we would have trouble. She said, "Lunch is on you." I said, "So be it." After each of us took a generous tray cafeteria style, we approached the cashier. He said, "It is all paid for." The student raised her eyes in surprise. The cashier explained, "That gentleman over there, the producer, said he took your classes and wanted to treat you and all your guests." I smiled, winked at the student, and said, "I'm sorry you didn't have the opportunity to receive the blessing of giving today. Apparently that kindness belongs to the gentleman over there." The student understood her wiles were thwarted.

Abundance is when you are supported and responded to by the unknown. It happens when your efforts are from the heart and done with innocence. That is the way of spirit. It has unlimited resources. They come from within and without in equal measure. This Breathwalk program attunes you to that reality within you. It uses an advanced breathing pattern, so be sure you read the description carefully in the Breathwalk guide. Build up to it after the more basic Breathwalks. If you master it gradually, it can change your life in amazing ways.

1. Awakener 1: Opening to Go
2. Align as you pace up to speed and scan your body.
3. a. Breathwalk 11: The Magnificent Lion (one-minute breath)

Vitality Intervals

1st Interval	Magnificent Lion	3 minutes
	Normal Breathing	2 minutes
2nd Interval	Magnificent Lion	5 minutes
	Normal Breathing	3 minutes
3rd Interval	Magnificent Lion	11 minutes
	Normal Breathing	5 minutes

b. Awakener 10: Being Present

4. Balance as you pace down and shift your focus for 2 minutes. Then do the triple balance stretch.

5. Innerwalk: Do an Innerwalk of your choice or stroll for a while as you enter a prayerful state and/or give prayers as you walk.

Awakener Exercises

Opening to Go

1. Breath priming for 1–3 minutes.

2. Stand straight with the feet placed shoulder width apart. Extend both arms in front. Interlace the fingers, palms together and curl them over the knuckles to form a hammerlock. With the elbows straight, begin a steady up-and-down pumping motion, lifting the arms up to a 60-degree angle and then bringing them down to an angle 60 degrees below the horizontal. Breathe through the nose, make your breath deep and smooth, and synchronize the breath with the arm movements. Inhale as you lift the arms up and exhale as they go down. Continue for 2–3 minutes. A good pace is 1 pump per second. To end, inhale with the arms up and hold for 5–10 seconds. Exhale and relax down.

3. Still standing, spread the legs slightly to form a steady base. Place the hands on the shoulders with the thumbs in back and fingers in front. Raise the elbows to the height of the shoulders. Begin to twist the head and torso left and right. Coordinate the movement with the breath inhaling as you twist left and exhaling as you twist right. Make sure to move the torso, arms, and head all together without "flapping" the elbows down or forward. Continue at a steady, smooth pace for 1–3 minutes. End with a deep inhale as you straighten and hold in the center for 5–10 seconds.

4. Stand with the legs together and begin rhythmical shoulder shrugs. Inhale as you lift both shoulders up and exhale as they drop down. Stay relaxed. Done properly, the "shrug" lifts the shoulders straight up and down. Do not squeeze the shoulders toward the neck. Create a steady pace of 5–8 shrugs per 5 seconds and continue for 1–3 minutes. To end, inhale, suspend the breath, and hold the shoulders up for 5 seconds. Then relax the arms, shake them out as you open, and close the fists.

Awakener 2

Hip and Spine Balance

1. Breath priming for 1–3 minutes.

2. Stand straight. Bring the hands to shoulder level, with the elbows relaxed by your sides. On each hand touch the tip of the index finger to the thumb tip. Stand in place and begin to march by lifting one knee to waist level as you inhale deeply and extend both arms straight up to the sky. Exhale as you bring the arms and the leg down. One cycle takes about 1 second. Repeat the motion with the opposite leg. Coordinate the breath, arms, and legs in a steady march that feels smooth and balanced. Mentally smile and keep your eyes fixed on the horizon. Continue for 1–3 minutes. To end, inhale deeply, stretch both arms up, hold for 5 seconds, and relax the arms down as you exhale.

3. Stand straight and spread your legs widely 2½–3 feet apart. Extend both arms out to the sides, parallel to the ground, with the palms facing down. Inhale deeply. As you exhale, bend forward and turn your torso to one side so you touch one hand to the toes of the opposite foot. Then inhale deeply back up into the original position. Immediately exhale and touch the other toes with the opposite hand. Emphasize smoothness of motion. Make sure to bend at the waist and do not throw your head and arms forward. Let the breath guide your motion. Set a comfortable and steady pace of about 3–4 cycles (touching each foot once) in 10 seconds. Continue for 1–3 minutes. To end, come up into the original position, inhale deeply, and hold for 5–10 seconds as you pull in the navel point gently. Then exhale and relax the arms.

4. Stand or sit comfortably with an erect spine. Interlace your fingers and touch the tips of the thumbs together. Place the hands in front of you, palms down, at the level of the navel point. The hands and forearms are parallel to the ground. Inhale as you raise the hands and forearms together up to the level of the throat. Then exhale as you quickly bring the hands and arms back down. Create a powerful, moderately fast pace. The breath is through the nose. The eyes may be open or closed and are focused at the brow point. Continue for 1–3 minutes. To end, inhale, hold the hands at the throat level, gently squeeze the root lock, and be perfectly still for 5–10 seconds. Exhale and relax the arms.

Awakener 3

Potency and Zeal

1. Breath priming for 1–3 minutes. (Breath of fire is recommended.)

2. Stand straight and spread your legs widely 2½–3 feet apart. Extend both arms out to the sides, parallel to the ground with the palms facing down. Inhale deeply. As you exhale, bend forward and turn your torso to one side so you touch one hand to the toes of the opposite foot. Then inhale deeply back up into the original position. Immediately exhale and touch the other toes with the opposite hand. Emphasize smoothness of motion. Make sure to bend at the waist, and do not throw your head and arms forward. Let the breath guide your motion. Set a comfortable and steady pace of about 3–4 cycles (touching each foot once) in 10 seconds. Continue for 1–3 minutes. To end, come up into the original position, inhale deeply, and hold for 5–10 seconds as you pull in the navel point gently. Then exhale and relax the arms.

3. Still standing, raise the arms over the head to the sky. Spread the fingers, palms facing up. Jump as high as you can 10–15 times in quick succession. Inhale a little as you jump up, exhale as you come down. Keep the arms up and stretch high when you jump! Then immediately do the next exercise.

4. Frog Pose: Squat down with your heels together and your knees spread. Reach down between your knees so your fingertips touch the ground. Your head is up, eyes level to the horizon, and the heels are up off the ground. Inhale and extend the legs so your buttocks rise up and your head

goes forward toward the knees. The arms will straighten as
your fingers stay on the ground. Exhale as you come back
into the squat with the head once again level. Repeat the
motion 10–15 times with a strong breath and a steady exercise pace. If you are advanced, you may increase the number of cycles up to a maximum of 108 squats. When done,
inhale up, and as you exhale stand all the way up.

Please note: If you have knee troubles and cannot squat, try
the following alternative. Stand straight with your arms out
in front, parallel to the ground. Exhale as you squat 1/3 to
1/2 of the way down. Inhale and stand straight. Repeat the
motion 10–15 times with a strong breath.

5. Archer Pose: Standing, turn slightly sideways and
extend one leg forward about 1 1/2–2 feet. Bend the front
knee forward over the toes. Stretch the other leg straight
back with the foot extended forward at a 45-degree angle.
Reach forward with the same arm as the front leg and
make a fist as if you were grasping a bow. With the other
hand imagine yourself grasping the bowstring and pull it all
the way back. Focus your eyes over the front hand to the
horizon. Fix your gaze without blinking. Begin a steady,
powerful breath of fire. Continue for 1–3 minutes. Then inhale, shift the front knee a little more forward, and hold the
breath in for 5–10 seconds. Stand up as you exhale. Then
switch to the opposite arms and legs and repeat the exercise. After you complete both sides, shake out legs and arms
for 10–15 seconds.

Awakener 4

Relax and Center

1. Breath priming for 1–3 minutes. Complete deep breathing is recommended. Focus at the brow point if you need to go within, center, and let go of things. Focus on the tip of the nose if you want to relax, gently energize, and become active later.

2. Star Pose: Stand straight and spread the legs wide. Extend both arms out to the sides, parallel to the ground with the palms facing up. Focus the eyes at the tip of the nose, or close them and focus at the brow point. Begin a slow complete deep breath. Inhale deeply; exhale completely, remembering to pull in the navel with the last bit of exhalation. Concentrate mentally on the feeling of the breath in the center of each palm. Sense the connection between your breath and the range of all life. Continue for 1–3 minutes. To end, inhale deeply, apply the root lock, and hold the breath for 5–10 seconds. Then relax the arms and breathe normally.

3. Stand straight with your legs together. Stretch both arms straight up over the head and bring the palms together. The elbows should be straight, with the arms hugging the ears. Close the eyes and roll them up to focus through the top of the head. Mentally imagine your posture, balanced and strong. Again begin a slow complete deep breath. Feel the flow of breath. As you inhale visualize light extending from the body into the world and universe. As you exhale imagine the universe contracting slightly, bringing a response to your bright flash of radiance. Continue for 1–3 minutes. To end, inhale deeply, hold 5–10 seconds. Exhale completely, hold the breath out, and apply the root lock; hold for 5–10 seconds. Then inhale and relax.

4. Stand or sit with a straight spine. Place the hands, palms together, at the center of the chest, with the fingers pointing up (as if you are praying). Inhale and extend the arms out to the sides, parallel to the ground. Keep the wrists bent at a 90-degree angle. (When fully extended, the hands look as though they are pressed against two walls with the fingers up.) Exhale completely as you bring them smoothly back to the center of the chest. Set a pace of 5–7 cycles every 15 seconds and continue for 1–3 minutes. To end, inhale with the arms held out, suspend the breath, and apply the root lock for 5–10 seconds. Then exhale and relax.

5. Stand or sit with a straight spine. Relax the shoulders and lift the chest slightly. Cross the hands, right hand over left, and place them on the center of the chest with palms against the chest. Begin complete deep breathing. As you inhale turn your head to the left. As you exhale turn your head to the right. Make the turns smooth and effortless. Do not strain at the extremes, instead relax the neck and shoulder muscles as you complete an inhale or exhale. Set a pace of 5–7 cycles per 15 seconds and continue for 1–3 minutes.

To end, inhale with your head straight and hold 5–10 seconds. Exhale completely, inhale, exhale, and suspend the breath out as you apply the root lock for 5–10 seconds. Relax the breath and take a moment to notice the increased sense of peacefulness and centering.

Awakener 5

New Lungs

1. Breath priming for 1–3 minutes.

2. **a.** Stand straight with the legs together. Balance equally on the two feet. Extend your arms straight out (no bend at the elbows) in front of you, parallel to the ground with the palms down. With each hand touch the tip of the little finger to the tip of the thumb, keep the other fingers straight but relaxed. Swing the arms in giant circles up and back over the head, then down in back, around, then forward and up. Inhale as you start to swing up and exhale as you start to swing around and forward. Make your swing full, relaxed, automatic, and strong. Continue for 2–3 minutes. Then inhale and stretch the arms straight up for 5–10 seconds. Proceed immediately to 2b.

2. **b.** Reverse the direction of the arm swing. Start by making fists of both hands and stretch your arms straight in front, parallel to the ground. Swing the arms down in front, up in back, and over the head. Keep the arms straight and swing them powerfully. Continue for 1 minute. To end, inhale with the arms stretched forward, tighten the fists, and hold for 5–10 seconds. Exhale and relax.

3. Stand or sit with a straight spine. Place the hands in front of the chest. Make the hands into a tepee by putting corresponding fingertips together, spreading the fingers slightly, and separating the palms. Begin making large circles, 1–2 feet in diameter, in front of the chest. Inhale deeply as you circle upward and then out, exhale as you go downward and then in. The shoulders move smoothly in smaller circles, supporting the motion of the hands. Continue for 1–3 minutes. Then inhale, suspend the breath, and press the fingertips together firmly in front of the heart center for 5–10 seconds. Exhale and relax.

4. Stand or sit with a straight spine. Put your hands on the shoulders, palms down, with the elbows out to the sides at shoulder height. Inhale and extend the arms out to the sides with the palms up. Exhale and bring them back to the shoulders. Inhale and stretch the arms straight up, palms facing each other. Exhale and bring the hands back to the shoulders. Create a fast, steady rhythm and match it with a strong breath. Continue for 1–3 minutes. To end, inhale, stretch the arms up, and hold for 5–10 seconds. Exhale and relax.

5. Sit with a straight spine. Stretch the arms out to the sides, parallel to the ground. Bend the arms up at the elbow to 90 degrees with the palms forward. Tilt the hands back at the wrist until the palms are facing up and the wrists are locked with the fingers pointing back. Hold this posture throughout the exercise.

Begin the following breath cycle: Inhale, exhale, inhale, exhale, inhale deeply, suspend the breath, apply the root lock, and hold as long as you are comfortable—say, 15–30 seconds.

Then exhale, inhale, exhale completely, pull in the navel, apply root lock, lift the diaphragm, and suspend the breath out as long as you can—say, 10–30 seconds.

Continue this cycle for 3 minutes. Develop this exercise so you can hold the breath for about 1 minute.

Awakener 6

Spinal Flex

1. Breath priming for 1–3 minutes. (The complete deep breath is my recommendation if you are working on spinal flexibility.)

2. Sit in a cross-legged posture with a straight spine. Grab your ankles or shins with both hands. Close the eyes and focus at the brow point. As you inhale lift the chest up and flex the spine forward, pulling the shoulders back gently. As you exhale flex the spine back and let the pelvis tip back naturally. Flex back and forth smoothly and steadily, keeping the head level. Continue for 1–2 minutes. To end, inhale, suspend the breath, apply root lock, and hold for 5–10 seconds. Exhale and relax.

3. Still sitting, grab your elbows and relax your arms, relaxed on the chest. Begin to twist your torso left and then right rapidly. Exhale as you swing to each side and inhale as you pass the center of the swing. If done correctly, this will develop into a natural breath of fire. Continue for 1–2 minutes. To end, inhale into the center and suspend the breath for 5–10 seconds. Exhale and relax.

4. Standing or sitting with a straight spine, put the hands at shoulder height with the palms facing forward and the elbows relaxed by the sides. Lock the index finger tip on top of the thumb tip. Inhale deeply and stretch both arms straight up. Exhale as you bring the elbows strongly down to the original position. Rapidly continue this up-and-down motion (8–15 cycles in 10 seconds) for 1–2 minutes. To end, inhale, stretch the arms straight up, and suspend the breath for 5 seconds. Exhale and relax.

5. Stand with the legs together. Place your hands on the hips and make wide circles with your torso. Circle forward as you inhale and back as you exhale. The motion should be balanced and smooth and not too fast. Continue for 1–2 minutes. To end, straighten the torso, inhale, and suspend the breath for 5 seconds. Exhale and relax.

6. Sit with your legs spread wide apart. Reach forward and grasp the toes. (If you can't reach that far, grasp the farthest point along the legs that is comfortable for you.) Hold the toes as you inhale and straighten up in the center. Exhale and bend at the waist over one leg. Inhale back up to the center and then exhale and bend down over the other leg. Continue this alternating side-to-side motion for 1–2 minutes. To end, inhale deep, continue to hold the toes as you stretch the spine up in the center and pull in the chin. Suspend the breath for 5–10 seconds and concentrate at the brow point. Exhale and relax. Then stand up and shake out your limbs and arms.

Awakener 7

Better Moods

1. Breath priming for 1–3 minutes. Since all the following exercises use a form of breath of fire, you might want to do complete deep breaths for balance and preparation.

2. Sit with a straight spine. Position the left hand to block the left nostril with the thumb. The other fingers point straight up with the palm facing right. Start a strong breath of fire through the right nostril. Remember to keep the inhale/exhale ratio equal. Continue for 1–3 minutes. To

end, inhale deeply, apply the root lock, and become per-fectly still for 5–15 seconds. Exhale and relax.

3. Stand or sit with an erect spine. Keep the eyes open and look to the horizon. Make fists of both hands. Begin to alternately "punch" with one fist, then the other. Together the hands create a pistonlike motion, with one arm pulling back to balance the other arm punching forward. The hands do not turn or twist. Exhale with each punch for-ward and punch rapidly so the breath becomes like a breath of fire. Continue for 1–3 minutes. To end, inhale, draw both elbows back, tighten the fists, apply the root lock, and sus-pend the breath for 5 seconds. Exhale and relax.

4. a. Stand or sit with an erect spine. Stretch both arms in front, parallel to the ground and each other. The palms are facing down. Start to crisscross the arms each time, al-ternating the arm that is on top. Move rapidly and syn-chronize the movement with a breath of fire. Exhale as the arms come together and crisscross. Inhale as they return to the parallel position. Continue for 1–2 minutes. Proceed immediately to 4b.

4. b. Raise the arms up to an angle of 60 degrees and continue the same crisscross motion with breath of fire for 1–2 more minutes. To end, inhale deep, stretch the arms out to a 60-degree angle, suspend the breath, and apply the root lock for 5–10 seconds. Exhale and relax.

5. Circles of fire. Stand straight with the legs together. Stretch the arms out to the sides, parallel to the ground with the palms facing forward. Spread the fingers of the hands very wide, so you can feel the webs stretch between them. Start tracing rapid circles with the arms (1–2 feet in diameter) as you begin the breath of fire. Coordinate the breath with the motion and continue for 1 minute.

Immediately inhale and close all the fingertips together

like a closed flower. Bring the fingertips to the shoulders, making sure to keep the elbows at shoulder height out to the sides. Hold the breath in for 5 seconds. Then exhale completely, suspend the breath out, and apply the root lock for 5–10 seconds. Inhale deeply, extend the arms back to the original position.

Repeat this entire exercise 1 or 2 more times.

Awakener 8

Pure Joy

1. Breath priming for 1–3 minutes.

2. Sit straight. Place elbows at your sides and slightly in front of the torso. The palms face forward with the fingers pointing up and the thumbs stretched straight out away from the hand. Keep the thumb out and straight throughout the exercise. In one complete motion twist the hands and curl the fingers down into the palms. (When this motion is complete your hands will be in fists with the palms facing toward your shoulders and the thumbs will have rotated so they are pointing away from each other.) Immediately rotate the hands back and extend the fingers. Continue this motion, creating a fast, steady rhythm for 3 full minutes. Coordinate the motion with a powerful cannon breath through the mouth. Your eyes should be fixed on the tip of the nose. To end, inhale and hold the hands steady with the palms facing forward for 10–30 seconds. Exhale and relax for 1 minute.

3. Sit straight with a straight spine and the chest lifted. Begin alternately pushing your arms out as if you are pushing something away from you. Push one hand out as you pull the other arm back along the side. The palms face forward with the fingers relaxed. Alternate quickly and coordinate the motion with a powerful cannon breath through the mouth. Keep the eyes open and fixed on the horizon. Continue for 3 minutes. To end, inhale and press one hand forward with the arm extended as you hold the other back. Tighten all the muscles and hold for 10–30 seconds. Exhale, inhale, and switch arms. Again tighten all the muscles and hold for 10–30 seconds. Exhale and relax for 1 minute.

4. Still sitting, relax your elbows down by your sides and extend forearms out to the side. Lift your elbows slightly away from your sides and angle the forearms so your hands end up at the level of the navel with the palms facing forward and the fingers relaxed.

Begin to move the hands and lower forearms in fast circles, as if you were trying to paddle backward. Coordinate the motion with a powerful cannon breath and continue for 3 minutes. To end, inhale deeply and suspend the breath for 10–30 seconds. Exhale and relax.

Awakener 9

Intuitively Right

1. Breath priming for 1–3 minutes.

2. Sit with a straight spine, or stand straight with the feet spread slightly to give you a firm base. This rhythmical exercise uses an 8-beat count to cycle smoothly through the following 8 steps. Please note that some steps involve a change in position while others constitute a complete motion that returns to the original position. In either case, each step counts as one beat. Proceed through each step in a precise, steady cadence.

Starting position: Place both palms facing each other about 6 inches apart in front of the chest. The fingertips point up with the wrists locked at a 90-degree angle. The fingers are straight, not relaxed. The elbows are lifted slightly as if you were about to push the hands together.

a. Smoothly extend the right arm fully out to the side, parallel to the ground, palm forward with the wrist straight. Quickly return to the starting position.
b. Smoothly extend the left arm fully out to the side, parallel to the ground, palm forward with the wrist straight. Quickly return to the starting position.
c. Extend both arms straight up with the palms facing toward each other and the fingers pointing toward the sky.
d. Return to the starting position.
e. Repeat a.
f. Repeat b.
g. Extend both arms out to the sides with the elbows straight and the palms facing forward.
h. Return to the starting position. Continue the sequence starting from a.

To end, inhale and hold the hands fixed in the starting position for 10–15 seconds. Exhale and then inhale deep as you stretch both hands up and hold for another 10 seconds. Exhale and relax. Beginners should practice this sequence for 3 minutes. Intermediate students can increase to 5 minutes, with advanced students increasing gradually to 11 minutes.

3. Stand with the feet shoulder width apart. Place your hands on your hips with your elbows out to the sides and back. Rotate your upper body around, forming large circles. Synchronize the motions of the torso and waist. Go at an easy pace that allows you to create full circles without getting dizzy. Continue for 2 minutes. To end, inhale as you straighten up in the center and then relax the breath.

4. Stand tall and place your hands on the waist. Come up on the balls of both feet and begin to alternately kick each foot forward and up. These are little kicks, and the knees remain straight. Create a rapid motion of about 2 kicks per second. Continue for 2 minutes as a beginner and 3 minutes if more practiced.

To create a great impact on your intuition and to add the force of that to your ability to communicate effectively, add the following primal sounds in an 8-beat rhythm to the above movement: HUM   DUM   HAR   HAR HAR   HAR   HUM   DUM.

This sequence of sounds plays your nerves like an instrument. The lips, diaphragm, and navel point are stimulated, and your nerves wake up and dance with you.

Awakener 10

Being Present

1. Breath priming for 1–3 minutes.

2. Stand straight. Extend the arms up and out to the sides to form 60-degree angles with the horizon. The wrists are straight and the palms face up with the fingers extended. Pull in the chin slightly so the neck is straight.

Begin a steady, powerful breath of fire and continue for 3 minutes. To end, inhale deeply and suspend the breath for 10 seconds. Exhale and relax as you let the arms down.

3. Stand straight and raise the arms up at your sides, parallel to the ground. Bend the elbows so the forearms point straight up, forming a 90-degree angle at the elbows. The palms face forward with the fingers pointing up. On each hand touch the tip of the index finger to the tip of the thumb. Hold this arm position steady and begin to twist your torso left and right. Swing your torso and arms as one unit. Synchronize the motion with the breath, inhaling as you twist to the left and exhaling as you twist to the right. Continue for 2 minutes. To end, inhale deep as you center the torso and suspend the breath for 10 seconds. Exhale as you relax the arms.

4. Repeat the following sequence of steps with a smooth, steady rhythm. One full cycle of four positions takes about 4 seconds.

Starting position: Stand straight and place your palms together at the center of the chest, with the fingers pointing up (prayer pose).

   a. Inhale deeply as you extend the arms out to your sides, parallel to the ground with the palms facing up.

   b. Exhale as you raise your arms up over the head so that your palms come together with the fingers pointing to the sky. Your elbows should hug the ears.

   c. Inhale as you return the arms back out to the sides as in position a.

   d. Exhale as you return to the starting position. Continue for 3 minutes.

5. Stand or sit with a straight spine. Feel for your pulse by placing the fingertips of your right hand on the under-side of the left wrist about 2 inches down from the thumb. Press just hard enough to feel the pulse. Close your eyes and concentrate on the qualities of the pulse. Is it jumpy, smooth, soft, strong, wavelike? Allow your breath to become very slow and meditative. Allow your awareness to expand until you can feel the pulse in your fingers, hands, torso, and the rest of the body. Become totally focused on the present moment and the rhythm of your own pulse. Let the breath become slower and longer as you feel the beat everywhere. Continue for 3–5 minutes.

Next open your eyes and look around as you keep the breath slow. Restrict no sensations. Hear, see, and feel everything. Continue for 2 more minutes, then relax.

Awakener 11

Letting Go

1. Breath priming for 1–3 minutes.
2. Stand straight. Extend both arms in front and with palms together interlace the fingers to form a hammerlock. With the elbows straight, begin a steady up-and-down pumping motion, lifting the arms up to a 60-degree angle and then bringing them down to an angle 60 degrees below the horizontal. Breathe through the nose, make your breath deep and smooth, and synchronize the breath with the arm movement. Inhale as you lift the arms up and exhale as they go down. Continue for 2–3 minutes. To end, inhale with the arms up and hold the position with breath suspended for 5–10 seconds. Exhale and relax down.

3. Stand straight and extend the arms straight out in front of you at the level of the heart. Keeping the elbows straight, place the right palm on the back of the left hand with both palms facing down. Open the fingers and interlace them slightly, making sure to keep all the fingers straight, not bent. Begin to alternately swing the arms left and right. Coordinate the motion with the breath, inhaling as you swing to the left and exhaling as you swing to the right. Set a steady pace and continue 2–3 minutes. To end, inhale deep as you center the torso, keeping the arms extended. Suspend the breath for 10 seconds. Exhale and relax.

4. Interlace your fingers and place the palms on your belly over the navel point. Focus your eyes down past the tip of the nose. Create a steady, powerful breath through a rounded mouth. Breathe so the inhale and exhale are exactly equal and not jerky or erratic. In this exercise the control of the flow of breath comes from the throat area, not the lips. Breathe this way for 1 minute. Then inhale and relax. Please note: If you get dizzy at all, be sure to stop. You may need to adjust your breath.

5. Sit in a cross-legged posture with a straight spine. Trace the following path with your hands. Begin with your hands resting over the knees and the palms facing up. Lift the arms upward by tracing a path in from the knees toward the centerline and up. When the hands are at the top of the circular path, they are above the head, out to the sides, with the palms facing toward each other. From that zenith the arms come down by going slightly out from the body and circling back onto the knees. When you lift the arms up do it forcefully and with speed. Your breath will automatically inhale a little. As the arms come down the breath will release. Keep this cycle going for 3 minutes. Advanced practitioners can go as long as 5 minutes. To end, inhale deep, stretch both arms up over your head, and stretch the spine up. Exhale and relax.

6. Still sitting, cross both hands over the heart center (right hand over left) with palms in toward the chest. Look down the nose. Repeat the mouth breathing described in exercise 4 for 1 minute. Then inhale, close the mouth, and roll your eyes up. Let the breath go and simply follow the natural flow of your breath for 1–3 minutes.

As you watch the flow of your breath, allow it to connect you to your own feeling of aliveness and being. Create a feeling of being as vast as an ocean. Let go of everything as you connect to your vastness. Sense everything, feel everything, and forgive everything.

Awakener 12

Loving Feelings

1. Breath priming for 1–3 minutes.

2. Stand or sit with an erect spine. Keep the eyes open and look to the horizon. Make fists of both hands. Begin to alternately "punch" with one fist, then the other. Together the hands create a pistonlike motion, with one arm pulling back to balance the other arm punching forward. The hands do not turn or twist. Exhale with each punch forward and punch rapidly so the breath becomes like a breath of fire. Continue for 2–3 minutes. To end, inhale, draw both elbows back, tighten the fists, apply the root lock, and suspend the breath for 5 seconds. Exhale and relax.

3. Stand straight, extend your arms out to the sides, and begin to make big circles with both arms at the same

time. Inhale as they come forward and up and exhale as they go back and down. Continue for 2 minutes. To end, inhale and stretch both arms straight up over your head. Exhale and relax.

4. Sit straight. Interlace your fingers with the thumb tips touching each other. Position the hands 4–6 inches in front of the chest with both palms facing down. Lift the elbows to the same level. Inhale as you lift the hands up to the level of the throat. Exhale as you sweep them down to the level of your navel. Keep the elbows and hands in one level line. Create a steady pumping motion with a powerful breath and continue for 3 minutes. To end, inhale, place the hands at the level of the heart, and suspend the breath for 10 seconds. Exhale and relax.

5. Stand or sit with a straight spine. Place the hands to the sides of the shoulders with your elbows by your sides and the palms facing forward. Close your eyelids halfway and fix your gaze downward. Begin to slowly inhale and exhale. Your breath should be equal on the inhale and exhale. Mentally repeat the following primal sound scale on both the inhale and exhale: SA TA NA MA SA TA NA MA.

Using the instructions from the chapter on finger magic, play the fingertips along with the mental sounds. Continue for 3–5 minutes.

6. Stand or sit with a straight spine. Block the right nostril gently with the index finger of the right hand and inhale slowly through your left nostril. Then exhale slowly through rounded lips. Match the duration of the inhale and exhale, with each one lasting about 10 seconds. Continue with this slow breathing pattern for 3 minutes. Then relax and follow the natural flow of your breath for another 2 minutes.

Breathwalk Patterns

Breathwalk 1

The Eagle • *Pattern: 4/4 Segmented Breath*

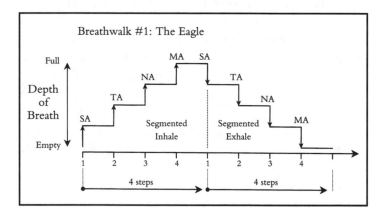

The Eagle uses a natural walking rhythm and an easy breath pattern. Simply coordinate your steps with your breath as you inhale through the nose in 4 segments and then exhale through the nose in 4 segments. Add the following primal sound scale:

Inhale and mentally recite	SA TA NA MA
Exhale and mentally recite	SA TA NA MA

Each syllable corresponds to a step and a segment of breath. To increase the sense of balance and evenness of mood, make sure to use finger magic.

Breathwalk 2

The Dove • ***Pattern: 8/8 Seqmented Breath***

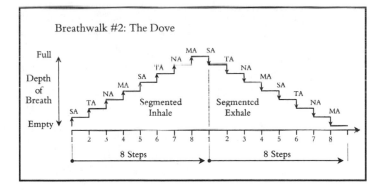

Breathwalk #2: The Dove

To perform the Dove, synchronize your steps with your breath as you inhale in 8 segments and exhale in 8 segments through the nose. The Dove is a natural deepening of the 4/4 segmented breath used in the Eagle and requires a little more attention to form. The Dove is usually done with a slightly slower walking pace than the Eagle. The impact is increased not by speed and effort, but by a focus on the depth and completeness of the breath. Focus on making the breath segments small so you don't fill up too soon on the inhale or run out of air too soon on the exhale. When exhaling, feel your upper chest and start the short exhales from there. Progressively contract the middle and then lower chest and consciously pull in the navel point on the last 2 or 3 exhales. The next inhale will begin automatically, where it should, at the navel point area. Add the following primal sound scale:

Inhale and mentally recite	SA TA NA MA NA MA	SA TA
Exhale and mentally recite	SA TA NA MA NA MA	SA TA

Each syllable corresponds to a step and segment of the breath. Use finger magic to deepen the healing impact and the sense of centeredness.

Breathwalk 3

The Hawk • *Pattern: 8/4 Segmented Breath*

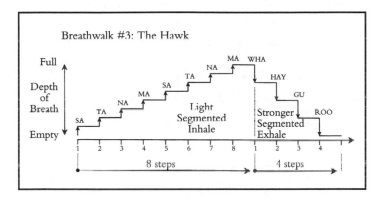

Breathwalk #3: The Hawk

The Hawk utilizes an uneven 8/4 segmented breath. Synchronize the steps with the breath as you inhale through the nose in 8 segments and then exhale through the nose in 4 segments. Inhalations should be light and equal. Exhalations are stronger to facilitate a complete exhale in 4 strokes.

As you establish the pattern the breath will become powerful and automatic. Add the following primal sound scales:

Inhale and mentally recite	SA TA NA MA SA TA NA MA
Exhale and mentally recite	WHA HAY GU ROO

Each syllable corresponds to a breath segment and a step.

Breathwalk 4

The Owl • *Pattern: 4/8 Segmented Breath*

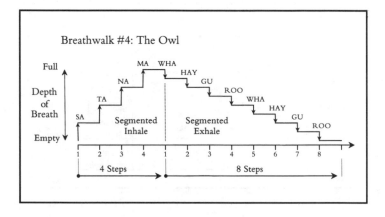

Breathwalk #4: The Owl

The Owl uses a 4/8 segmented breath. Synchronize your steps with your breath as you inhale in 4 equal segments through the nose and then exhale in 8 equal segments through the nose. To "flow" with this rhythm, emphasize the inhales and pay attention to the natural tendency to exhale too quickly. A good program for mastering the Owl is to begin with 3-minute intervals followed by 1 minute of regular walk. Continue for 20 minutes. Once the breath pattern feels very comfortable, gradually increase the intervals to 5 minutes of Owl followed by 2 minutes of normal and then finally to 10 and 3. The effects of this Breathwalk build slowly over 5–10 minutes. Once you can properly regulate the breath so it is smooth, the wonders of this walk become yours. To heighten the impact, use the following primal sound scales:

Inhale and mentally recite	SA TA NA MA
Exhale and mentally recite	WHA HAY GU ROO
	WHA HAY GU ROO

Each syllable corresponds to a segment of breath and a step.

Breathwalk 5

The Tiger • *Pattern: 4/4 (or 8/8) Complete Deep Breath*

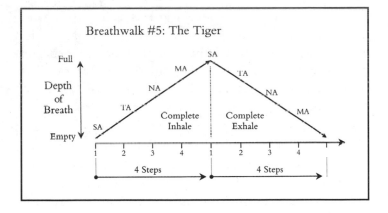

Breathwalk #5: The Tiger

The Tiger is performed with a 4/4 or 8/8 complete deep breath that maintains an equal inhale/exhale ratio. Begin this practice with 4/4. As you inhale slowly and steadily, take 4 steps and then slowly and steadily exhale over the next 4 steps. It is important to take a full complete deep breath. There is a tendency to be satisfied with a shallow breath or one that doesn't push out enough air. To avoid this, pay attention to the end of both the inhale and the exhale. For the last part of the inhale remember to consciously relax the shoulders and lift the chest a bit without tightening the stomach. This lets the upper lungs expand. For the last part of the exhale you must consciously expel the breath by pulling the belly and navel in toward the spine. As you acclimate to the pattern, adjust your stride length to the level of effort and the depth of breath you want. You should not feel "winded" but rather "open and aerated."

To increase the impact of this Breathwalk, try switching to an 8/8 complete deep breath. It may be difficult to start directly at 8/8, so take it easy and increase slowly through 5/5, 6/6, and 7/7. Once you are accustomed to the 8/8, increase your stride to a level slightly past your normal comfort zone to get the full training effects. The Tiger at 4/4 or 8/8 can be practiced over varied and challenging terrain. For the Tiger use one of the two following primal sound scales.

Option 1
Inhale and mentally recite   SA TA NA MA
Exhale and mentally recite   SA TA NA MA

Each syllable corresponds to 1 step. For the longer 8/8 pattern simply repeat the primal sound scales twice. This primal sound scale will give balance and a sense of focused attention.

Option 2
Inhale and mentally recite   SA TA NA MA
Exhale and mentally recite   WHA HAY GU ROO

Once again each syllable corresponds to 1 step, and for the longer 8/8 pattern simply repeat the primal sound scales twice. This scale pattern will help create a great sense of relaxation and steadfastness.

The Cheetah • ***Pattern: 8/4 Complete Deep Breath***

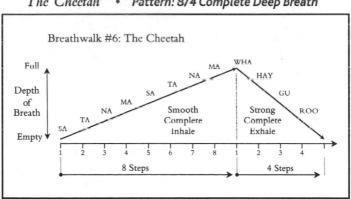

The Cheetah is performed with an 8/4 complete deep breath. Inhale completely as you take 8 steps and then exhale completely as you take 4 steps. Start the inhale smoothly, without a gasp or a fast intake, and keep the flow of the inhale even throughout the 8 steps. Remember that a complete deep breath begins by first relaxing the belly. Near the end of the inhale relax the shoulders and lift the upper chest a little to get in the last bit of air. The exhale takes half the time of the inhale. You will need to consciously pull in the navel to expel all the breath. Whenever you practice a nonequal ratio breath like the Cheetah, begin gradually with reasonable intervals, like 3–5 minutes of Breathwalk followed by 2 minutes of normal walking. When the pattern is established increase the time to 10 minutes of Breathwalk and 3 minutes of normal walking. Use the following primal sound scales:

Inhale and mentally recite	SA TA NA MA SA TA NA MA
Exhale and mentally recite	WHA HAY GU ROO

Each syllable corresponds to a step.

The Lion • *Pattern: 4/4/4 (or 8/8/8) Complete Deep Breath*

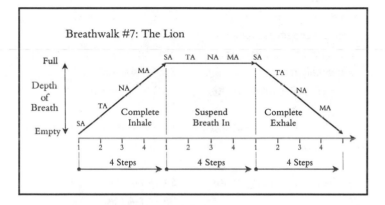

Breathwalk #7: The Lion

This is a very powerful breath pattern and should be attempted only after practicing some of the other Breathwalks. The Lion divides the breath cycle into three phases: inhale, hold, and exhale. To perform it, inhale steadily through the nose as you take 4 steps, suspend the breath as you take 4 steps, and then exhale evenly for 4 steps. The breath suspension is accomplished by lifting the chest a little rather than locking the throat and neck.

The extra phase of suspending the breath is natural and increases the utilization of oxygen in your system. It can be overdone if you are not healthy or if you push the time too long at first. Build the practice in a way that is comfortable. Start with a 3-minute interval of Breathwalk followed by 2 minutes of normal walking. Increase intervals slowly to 5 minutes breath, 3 minutes normal; then up to 10 minutes breath, 3 minutes normal; and finally take it to 10 minutes breath, 5 minutes normal with a good stride. Repeat this last cycle 1–4 times for a fantastic boost to health and well-being. Once you are comfortable with the 4/4/4 pattern, increase it to an 8/8/8. The primal sound scales used are dependent on which walking pattern you choose. For the 4/4/4 pattern:

Inhale and mentally recite	SA TA NA MA
Suspend the breath and mentally recite	SA TA NA MA
Exhale and mentally recite	SA TA NA MA

When you go to the longer 8/8/8 pattern use the following scale:

Inhale and mentally recite	SA TA NA MA
	SA TA NA MA
Suspend the breath and and mentally recite	SA TA NA MA
	WHA HAY GU ROO
Exhale and mentally recite	WHA HAY GU ROO
	WHA HAY GU ROO

In both instances each syllable corresponds to 1 step.

Breathwalk 8

The Blissful Eagle • ***Pattern: 4/4 Segmented/
Whispered Breath***

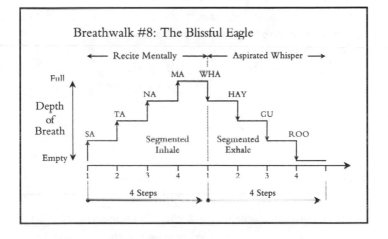

Breathwalk #8: The Blissful Eagle

The Blissful Eagle uses a 4/4 segmented breath pattern. Inhale through the nose in 4 breath segments and exhale in 4 segments through the mouth as you whisper a primal sound scale. Use the following primal sound scales:

As you inhale mentally recite	SA TA NA MA
Exhale with a strong	
aspirated whisper	WHA HAY GU ROO

Each syllable corresponds to a segment of breath and a step. The effects of this Breathwalk build rapidly if you emphasize the strong aspirated whisper on the exhale. To increase the power of this, make sure to use finger magic.

You can enhance the impact by creating an internal

feeling and image of bliss. Think on the sound WHA of un-limited ecstasy, as in "Wow!" As you recite it lift the eyes slightly to the horizon and allow a smile to come in the eyes. On HAY feel that ecstasy present in the here and now in your heart. On GU and ROO realize that this experience uplifts and teaches with its sense of vastness. This Innerwalk matches and enhances the psychoactive impact of the pattern in the breath and primal sounds.

Breathwalk 9

The Intuitive Dove • **Pattern: 8/8 Segmented/ Whispered Breath**

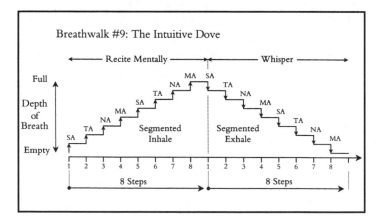

Breathwalk #9: The Intuitive Dove

To perform the Intuitive Dove, synchronize your steps with your breath as you inhale through your nose in 8 equal segments and then exhale in segments out through the mouth as you whisper a primal sound scale. For this Breathwalk use the following primal sound scale:

Inhale and mentally recite	SA TA NA MA	SA TA
	NA MA	
Exhale and whisper	SA TA NA MA	SA TA
	NA MA	

Each syllable corresponds to a segment of breath and a step. The whisper is done from midmouth and lips with the throat relaxed. You are whispering not to be quiet, but rather to stimulate the energy reflex points in the mouth. As you whisper listen to what you are saying. Put conscious intention behind your words and imagine you are communicating to yourself. Consciously speaking and using your volition creates a different impact from halfhearted or sleepy repetition. It is easy to catch the rhythm of this Breathwalk if you emphasize the first SA slightly. You may find it helpful to pull in the navel point with the last MA so you are ready to begin the inhales keeping the rhythm naturally.

Breathwalk 10

The Radiant Hawk • **Pattern: 8/4 Segmented/ Whispered Breath**

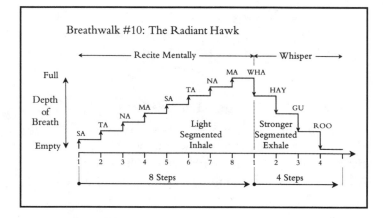

Breathwalk #10: The Radiant Hawk

The Radiant Hawk uses an 8/4 segmented/whispered breath pattern. Inhale in 8 segments through the nose and then exhale through the mouth in 4 segments as you whisper a primal sound scale. The segmented inhales should be equal and light. With only 4 steps to exhale, it needs to be done more forcefully so that the breath is completely out at the start of the next cycle of segmented inhales. Once you set this pattern, the breath becomes automatic and will carry you along with a sense of momentum and strength. Practicing longer intervals directs more reserve energy to your nervous system and gives added radiance to your personality projection. Use the following primal sound scales:

Inhale and mentally recite	SA TA NA MA SA TA NA MA
Exhale with a whisper	WHA HAY GU ROO

Each syllable corresponds to a segment of breath and a step.

Breathwalk 11

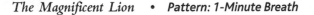

The Magnificent Lion • *Pattern: 1-Minute Breath*

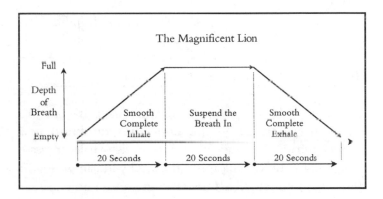

The Magnificent Lion uses a 1-minute breath pattern. The breath ratio is given in terms of time instead of steps or segments. Inhale slowly for 20 seconds using a complete deep breath, suspend the breath in as you walk steadily for 20 seconds, and then exhale slowly for 20 seconds. Remember to gradually pull in the navel for a complete exhale. Use either of the two following primal sound scales:

Breathwalk

Option 1
Simply focus on the gentle sound of your breath, your feet,
and nature.

Option 2
Inhale and mentally recite   SA TA NA MA
Suspend the breath and
mentally recite   WHA HAY GU ROO
Exhale and mentally recite   SA TA NA MA

The number of repetitions will vary according to your
pace and stride. An ideal combination for many people is
to inhale and walk at a pace so that you repeat the scale 8
times on the inhale, 8 times on the suspension, and 8 times
on the exhale. To enhance your experience, promote a feeling of vast openness and blessing, mentally recite WHA
HAY GU ROO as you suspend the breath.

Note: Build up to this practice gradually. It's good to
start with a shorter breath duration. Time your breath to 5
seconds inhale/5 seconds hold/5 seconds exhale. Increase
your walking time using this ratio until you can go for 15
minutes comfortably. Then increase the time a little. Try for
10 seconds inhale/10 seconds hold/10 seconds exhale.
Once again build up the time to 15 minutes comfortably.
Then increase the time a few seconds repeatedly until you
reach the goal of 20 seconds inhale/20 seconds hold/20
seconds exhale, and it becomes comfortable. At this level
begin with 3 minutes in intervals. Build to 5 minutes at a
time. Incrementally take it up to 11 minutes at once. Then
the magnificence comes through! The doubtless strength of
your spirit shines and heals.

Resources

For more information about Breathwalk, visit our website at www.Breathwalk.com. There you will find resources, inspiration, and products to enhance and refine your Breathwalk experience. Breathwalk instructor training programs are available.

There is a set of audio cassette tapes to guide you through four of the most popular Breathwalks for energy, clarity, mood elevation, and relaxation. Call 1–888–8BR–WALK or 781–237–9587 to order.

To correspond with Gurucharan Khalsa, send letters to

Khalsa Consultants, Inc.
18 Grove Street   Suite #5
Wellesley, MA   02482

For information about Yogi Bhajan, Kundalini yoga, and meditation visit the website www.yogibhajan.com or call the 3HO Foundation at 888–346–2420 or 505–753–6341 ext. 121.

To correspond with Yogi Bhajan, send letters to:

Yogi Bhajan
Rt. 2 Box 132D
Espanola, NM   87532

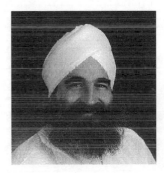

GURUCHARAN SINGH KHALSA, PH.D., is an expert on the mind, a yogi, psychotherapist, teacher, and writer. He is president of a business consulting firm, Khalsa Consultants, Inc., and has taught kundalini yoga with Yogi Bhajan for over thirty years. He lives in Millis, Massachusetts.

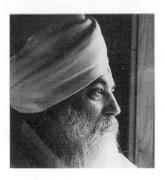

YOGI BHAJAN, PH.D., is a Master of kundalini and tantric yoga. He is the spiritual leader of the Sikh religion in the Western Hemisphere. He inspired the creation of the family of Golden Temple natural products, including Yogi Tea and Peace Cereals. He lives in Espanola, New Mexico.